An Illustrated Guide to Infection Control

Kathleen Motacki, MSN, RN, BC, Associate Clinical Professor at Saint Peter's College School of Nursing, Jersey City, New Jersey. She is a referral liaison at Children's Specialized Hospital, New Brunswick, New Jersey. She holds board certification in pediatric nursing from the American Nurses Credentialing Center (ANCC). She has recently been appointed to the ANCC Pediatric Content Expert Panel. She is Vice-President for Saint Peter's College for Mu-Theta-at-Large Chapter, Sigma Theta Tau International Nursing Honor Society. Professor Motacki obtained her BSN and MSN from Kean University, Union, New Jersey. She has published a continuing nursing education series for contact hours, "Safe Patient Handling in Pediatrics" in the *Journal of Pediatric Nursing*. Her book publications include *Nursing Delegation and Management of Patient Care* Mosby/Elsevier, *The Illustrated Guide to Safe Patient Handling and Movement*, Springer Publishing. She has presented the Sigma Theta Tau International Nursing Honor Society Biennium and was the keynote speaker at the Founders Day for the New Jersey Consortium of Chapters. She is a nurse philanthropist, and her volunteer efforts include: Our Lady of Fatima Rehabilitation Center in Liberia, Africa; Children's Specialized Hospital, New Brunswick, and the Sierra-Leone School of Nursing in Sierra-Leone Africa.

Neeta Bahal O'Mara, PharmD, BCPS, is a board-certified Pharmacotherapy Specialist and is licensed in New Jersey and Pennsylvania. She is presently employed as a consultant at Coldstream Consulting Company in Skillman, New Jersey, as a Clinical Pharmacist at Dialysis Clinic Inc. in North Brunswick, New Jersey, as a Drug Information Consultant at Pharmacist's Letter/Prescriber's Letter, Stockton, California, and as Associate Editor for Jones and Bartlett Learning for the Pocket Pharmacopoeia, Sudbury, Massachusetts. Her past experience was as a clinical pharmacist and family practice specialist at Methodist Hospital of Indiana in Indianapolis and Assistant Professor of Pharmacy Practice at Butler University, Indianapolis, Indiana. Dr. Bahal O'Mara was a Fellow in Pediatric Pharmacotherapy at the Wexner Institute for Pediatric Research / Ohio State University, Columbus, Ohio. She received her Doctor of Pharmacy from the Medical College of Virginia, Richmond, and her Bachelor of Science in Pharmacy from the Philadelphia College of Pharmacy and Science, Philadelphia, Pennsylvania.

Her professional affiliations include The American College of Clinical Pharmacy, the American Society of Hospital Pharmacists, the New Jersey Pharmaceutical Association, Rho Chi Pharmaceutical Honor Society, and the Kappa Epsilon Professional Pharmaceutical Fraternity. She has received many honors and awards, including Faculty of the Year from Family Practice Residency, Methodist Hospital. She has numerous areas of research experience, is widely published in peer-reviewed journals, and has authored several book chapters.

Toros Kapoian, MD, FAACP, is a Clinical Associate Professor of Medicine at the University of Medicine and Dentistry, Robert Wood Johnson Medical School in New Brunswick, New Jersey. He has specialty training in Kidney Transplantation and Clinical Hypertension. He serves as the Medical Director of the Kidney Center of New Jersey, Robert Wood Johnson University Hospital, and at the Dialysis Clinic, Inc. (DCI) facilities in North Brunswick and at Madison Center, where he also directs the Infection Control and Prevention Program. Dr. Kapoian is President of the Board of Trustees of the TransAtlantic Renal Council and serves on the Board of Trustees of the End Stage Renal Disease Network for New Jersey, Puerto Rico, and the Virgin Islands. He has expertise in both state and federal regulations pertaining to the care of patients with chronic kidney disease and teaches a structured approach to all aspects of quality assurance performance improvement, including infection control and prevention to nurses and health care providers alike.

An Illustrated Guide to Infection Control

- Kathleen Motacki, MSN, RN, BC
- Neeta Bahal O'Mara, PharmD, BCPS
- Toros Kapoian, MD, FAACP

SPRINGER PUBLISHING COMPANY
New York

Springer Publishing Company, LLC
11 West 42nd Street
New York, NY 10036
www.springerpub.com

Acquisitions Editor: Allan Graubard
Senior Production Editor: Diane Davis
Cover Design: Steven Pisano
Composition: Apex CoVantage

ISBN: 978-0-8261-0560-8
E-book ISBN: 978-0-8261-0561-5

11 12 13 14/5 4 3 2 1

The author and the publisher of this Work have made every effort to use sources believed to be reliable to provide information that is accurate and compatible with the standards generally accepted at the time of publication. Because medical science is continually advancing, our knowledge base continues to expand. Therefore, as new information becomes available, changes in procedures become necessary. We recommend that the reader always consult current research and specific institutional policies before performing any clinical procedure. The author and publisher shall not be liable for any special, consequential, or exemplary damages resulting, in whole or in part, from the readers' use of, or reliance on, the information contained in this book. The publisher has no responsibility for the persistence or accuracy of URLs for external or third-party Internet Web sites referred to in this publication and does not guarantee that any content on such Web sites is, or will remain, accurate or appropriate.

Library of Congress Cataloging-in-Publication Data

Motacki, Kathleen.
    An illustrated guide to infection control / Kathleen Motacki, Neeta Bahal O'Mara, Toros Kapoian.
        p. ; cm.
    Includes bibliographical references and index.
    ISBN 978-0-8261-0560-8 (alk. paper)
1. Infection—Prevention. 2. Nosocomial infections. 3. Communicable diseases—Nursing. I. O'Mara, Neeta Bahal. II. Kapoian, Toros. III. Title.
    [DNLM: 1. Infection Control—Nurses' Instruction. WC 195]
    RA761.M68   2010
    616.9—dc22   2010032176

Special discounts on bulk quantities of our books are available to corporations, professional associations, pharmaceutical companies, health care organizations, and other qualifying groups.

If you are interested in a custom book, including chapters from more than one of our titles, we can provide that service as well.

For details, please contact:
Special Sales Department, Springer Publishing, Company, LLC
11 West 42nd Street. 15th Floor, New York, NY 10036-8002
Phone: 877-687-7476 or 212-431-4370; Fax: 212-941-7842
Email: sales@springerpub.com

Printed in the United States of America by Hamilton Printing.

To my loving family:
  my husband, Robert;
  my son Robert;
  my lovely daughter, Lisa;
  my son John;
  and to Edward Motacki, my father-in-law;
  Irene Motacki, my mother-in-law;
  Ted Tatarek, my uncle; and
  Brian Motacki, my brother-in-law.

—Kathleen Motacki

To my loving family:
  Ed, Sean, Evan, and Neena.

—Neeta Bahal O'Mara

Contents

Contributors

Garletha Allen, RN, MSN, CNN   Nurse Manager, Dialysis Clinic, Inc., Monroe, New Jersey

Mary Jo Assi, MS, RN, APRN, BC, AHN-BC   Director: Advanced Practice Nursing, The Valley Hospital, Ridgewood, New Jersey

Kathleen A. Bivens, RN, CNN   Area Director of Nursing, Dialysis Clinic, Inc., North Brunswick, New Jersey

Lisa Bross Gajary, RN   Area Education Coordinator, Dialysis Clinic, Inc., North Brunswick, New Jersey

Kathleen Burke, PhD, RN   Assistant Dean in Charge of Nursing Programs, Professor of Nursing, Ramapo College of New Jersey, Mahwah, New Jersey

Beverly S. Karas-Irwin, MS, MSN, RN, NP-C   Director: Clinical Partnerships, Nursing Programs, The Valley Hospital, Ridgewood, New Jersey

Victor de la Cruz, RN   Vascular Access Coordinator, Dialysis Clinic, Inc., North Brunswick, New Jersey

Laura Kolmos, RN, HCS-D, COS-C   Medical Review Coder/Infection Control, Valley Home Care, Ridgewood, New Jersey

Patricia Mechan, PT, MPH, CCS   Consulting, Education & Clinical Services Manager, Guldmann, Inc., Belmont, Massachusetts

Lisa Marie Motacki, BA   Full-time Graduate Student, Caldwell College, Caldwell, New Jersey

Nicole A. Murad, RN, APN-C   Advanced Practice Nurse/Clinical Quality Specialist, Patient Care Services, The Valley Hospital, Ridgewood, New Jersey

Laura Murphy, RNC, MSN, WHNP-BC   Clinical Instructor at Valley Hospital (Ridgewood, New Jersey) for Ramapo College (Mahwah, New Jersey) Nursing Students; New York University Fertility Center, New York, New York; Greenwich Fertility and Invitro Fertilization Center, Greenwich, Connecticut

Reviewers

Dean Ann Tritak, RN, EdD   Dean of Nursing, Saint Peter's College, School of Nursing, Jersey City, New Jersey

Professor Lisa Garsman, MS, FNP, B-C   Director, BSN Program, Saint Peter's College, School of Nursing, Jersey City, New Jersey

Foreword

Infection control is a topic of exceptional importance for nurses, patients, and hospital or health care facility staff. With antibiotic-resistant infections at high levels, the student and new practicing nurse must be well-educated on infection control. It is vitally important to keep our patients and our nursing personnel free from nosocomial infections. Not only must nurses know how to keep patients free from such infections, they must know how to protect themselves from them as well, especially in high-risk areas: from dialysis units to operating rooms and trauma units. This guidebook gives you the knowledge to do just that in a variety of settings.

In addition, because health care facilities are environments of ever-increasing legislation and regulation, there is the need for more, not less, data on infections, along with associated reports. Taken together with the effects of the economic downturn, it is clear that most of us are asked to do more with less and are expected to provide a high standard of care with near-zero rates of infection. Whether this equates with an increase in staffing hours, loss of valuable resources, or limitations on reimbursement, the challenge is real. Certainly, the so-called superbugs complicate issues in terms of antibiotic resistance. Their ability to spread to ill patients has caused hospital wards to close, and in certain instances, they have caused patient death. We have to think smarter and do better. Remaining at the cutting edge of infection control and prevention requires not only new products to decrease infection rates but also the knowledge, skills, and mindset to be proactive against infection on a daily basis.

—Suresh K. Gupta, MD, F. CAP
Medical Director of Pathology and Laboratory Services
East Orange General Medical Center
East Orange, New Jersey
Clinical Assistant Professor of Laboratory Medicine and Pathology
UMDNJ Medical School
Newark, New Jersey

—Santosh Gupta, RN
Medical Coordinator
Franciscan Sisters,
Tenafly, New Jersey

Preface

An Illustrated Guide to Infection Control educates student nurses and new practicing nurses on effective infection control measures. Nursing textbooks, of course, cover infection control at the sophomore, junior, and senior levels. This book incorporates all of the levels of nursing into one book and includes basic infection control along with specialty area–specific infection control measures.

The book is designed for nursing students and beginning level RNs to help them develop a practical understanding of infection control issues as they relate to many different areas of health care. As a guide, the book is unique in that the contents cover infection control from basic handwashing to the exposure control plan, and everything in between. As health care providers we must act now to prevent hospital-acquired infections and decrease the number of infections in all health care settings. Thus, clinicians and educators who are experts in their fields have contributed to this book. The chapter writers discuss ways to protect patients, their families, visitors, volunteers, and health care providers from infection. Of course, superbugs also pose a great danger to patients, and we must be vigilant in our practices to prevent these hard-to-treat infections. The student nurse and beginning level nurse must be aware of the environment of care and as it relates to infection control. Indeed, infection control is everyone's responsibility. The clinical areas of expertise discussed include: acute care, physician's offices, labor and delivery, dialysis, and TB control, to name a few. There are pre-test and post-test questions for each chapter. The answers are included in the back of the book.

Infection control is everyone's responsibility. Infection-control committees and education specialists are challenged daily to make health care facilities safe for the patient, families, employees, visitors, and volunteers.

We know that you will come away from reading this book with information that you will use on a daily basis in your practice settings.

Acknowledgments

I am indebted to Dr. Toros Kapoian and Dr. Neeta Bahal O'Mara for agreeing to take on this project with me and for their lead on the contents of this book. It is because of their clinical, writing, and editing expertise that this book was possible. Their knowledge and expertise has made this book an excellent and exceptional resource for student nurses and for clinicians in a wide variety of health care fields. Thank you to Valley Hospital for allowing us to use your facility for excellent photography and staff input, and to the Dialysis Clinic, Inc., North Brunswick, New Jersey, and to Valley Hospital, Ridgewood, New Jersey, and their employees, the chapter writers, for agreeing to participate in this important and unique project. It is because of the writers' clinical expertise from Valley Hospital and Dialysis Clinic, Inc. that this book will be unique and current in a variety of different specialties. They have made the contents of this book an asset to student nurses and clinicians.

Thank you to the reviewers, Dr. Ann Tritak and Professor Lisa Garsman, from Saint Peter's College, Jersey City, New Jersey; it was crucial to have this book peer-reviewed. Thank you Daniel Hedden for your excellent photography work and to John Motacki for your assistance as our "model," allowing us to obtain excellent pictures. Thank you, Lisa Motacki, for your assistance with references and permissions, and to Dawn K. Harley, Trademark Paralegal and Permissions Coordinator Becton, Dickinson and Company. Thank you to the staff at Springer Publishing for your unending patience in bringing this publication to fruition: Elizabeth Stump, Assistant Editor; Diane Davis, Senior Production Editor; Rose Mary Piscitelli, Senior Production Editor; and Joanne Jay, Vice President, Production and Manufacturing; and to Laura Stewart, Project Manager, Apex Content Solutions.

Finally, I would like to thank my family for their unending support in my career endeavors and philanthropy work.

—*Kathleen Motacki*

Thank you to my co-editors for all of their hours of work to make a great book! And thank you to my husband, Ed, and children, Sean, Evan, and Neena, for being so understanding while I worked on the book.

—*Neeta Bahal O'Mara*

Basic Infection Control

This chapter includes topics on hand hygiene, proper hand-washing techniques, and the use of alcohol-based hand sanitizers. The barriers to proper hand hygiene are reviewed. The content differentiates between standard, airborne, droplet, and contact precautions. The Centers for Disease Control and Prevention guidelines regarding basic infection control are reviewed. There is discussion on caring for the immune-compromised patient. Finally, standard precautions and transmission-based precautions are discussed.

OBJECTIVES

1. Explain the importance of hand hygiene.
2. Describe proper hand-washing technique.
3. Discuss the use of alcohol-based hand sanitizers.
4. List some of the barriers to proper hand hygiene.
5. Differentiate between standard, airborne, droplet, and contact precautions.

PRE-TEST QUESTIONS

1-1. Appropriate hand hygiene can:
   a. Increase the risk of mortality
   b. Increase the rate of nosocomial infections
   c. Prevent the transmission of microorganisms
   d. Increase costs of health care–associated infections
1-2. Hands must always be washed with soap and water:
   a. When the hands are visibly dirty
   b. After contact with a patient's intact skin
   c. Before caring for patients with severe neutropenia or other forms of severe immunosuppression
   d. Before removing gloves

1-3. Which of the following is TRUE regarding hand washing?
    a. The water should be hot
    b. Hands and forearm should be kept higher than elbows during washing
    c. Hands should be washed for a minimum of 60 seconds
    d. Hands should be dried thoroughly from fingers to wrists and forearms with paper towel, single-use cloth, or warm air dryer

1-4. Which of the following is TRUE regarding the use of alcohol-based hand gels?
    a. Apply an ample amount of product to completely cover both hands
    b. Rub hands together, covering all surfaces of hands and fingers with antiseptic
    c. Rub hands together for several minutes until alcohol is dry
    d. If gloves are to be used, put gloves on while hands are still wet from the gel

1-5. Which of the following infectious precautions should be applied to a foreign-born national who is currently incarcerated and is being evaluated in the emergency department for fever, weight loss, pleuritic chest pain, and cough productive of bloody secretions of more than 3 weeks duration?
    a. Standard precautions
    b. Contact precautions
    c. Droplet precautions
    d. Airborne precautions

Hand hygiene is the single most effective way to prevent infections and disease transmission. It reduces the risks of microorganism transmission to patients while reducing the potential for health care worker (HCW) colonization or infection caused by organisms acquired from the patient. Hand hygiene reduces morbidity, mortality, and costs associated with health care–associated infections (HAI). Hand hygiene should be performed before and after patient care, whenever there may be contact with environmental surfaces that may be contaminated with blood or body fluids or are in the immediate vicinity of patients, before leaving or returning to a clinical area, after glove removal, and after performing personal hygiene such as applying make-up, blowing your nose, or using the bathroom (The Centers for Disease Control and Prevention [CDC], 2002).

The CDC guidelines for hand hygiene in *Health-Care Settings* (2002) recommend the following indications for hand washing and hand antisepsis:

1. When hands are visibly dirty or contaminated with proteinaceous material or are visibly soiled with blood or other body fluids, wash hands with either an antimicrobial or non-antimicrobial soap and water.
2. If hands are not visibly soiled, use either an antimicrobial soap and water or alcohol-based hand rub for routinely decontaminating hands in all other clinical situations such as:
    a. Before having direct contact with patients
    b. Before donning sterile gloves when inserting a central intravascular catheter

 c. Before inserting indwelling urinary catheters, peripheral vascular catheters, or other invasive devices that do not require a surgical procedure

 d. After contact with a patient's intact skin (e.g., when taking a pulse or blood pressure, and lifting a patient)

 e. After contact with body fluids or excretions, mucous membranes, nonintact skin, and wound dressings if hands are not visibly soiled

 f. If moving from a contaminated-body site to a clean-body site during patient care

 g. After contact with inanimate objects (including medical equipment) in the immediate vicinity of the patient

 h. After removing gloves

3. Before eating and after performing acts of personal hygiene such as using a restroom, applying make-up, or blowing your nose, wash hands with either an antimicrobial or non-antimicrobial soap and water.

4. Wash hands with either an antimicrobial or non-antimicrobial soap and water if exposure to *Bacillus anthracis* or *Clostridium difficile* is suspected or proven.

 a. The physical action of washing and rinsing hands under such circumstances is recommended because alcohols, chlorhexidine, iodophors, and other antiseptic agents have poor activity against spores.

Microorganisms associated with HAI are found both within skin and soft tissue infections (SSI) as well as normal looking, intact patient skin. Given that people shed more than one million skin cells each day, both the patient and their immediate environment (room, furniture, bed, linens, gowns, etc.) are potential sources for the transmission of HAIs. This can occur if an HCW's hands become contaminated with microorganisms that are able to survive, *and* if their hands are not decontaminated and they touch another patient or item in the patient's vicinity (CDC, 2002).

Sequence of events for the transmission of health care–associated pathogens via the hands of HCWs:

- Organisms present on the patient's skin, or that have been shed onto inanimate objects in close proximity to the patient, must be transferred to the hands of HCWs.
- These organisms must then be capable of surviving for at least several minutes on the hands of personnel.
- Next, hand washing or hand antisepsis by the worker must be inadequate or omitted entirely, or the agent used for hand hygiene must be inappropriate.
- Finally, the contaminated hands of the caregiver must come in direct contact with another patient, or with an inanimate object that will come into direct contact with the patient.

Hand washing is a vigorous, brief rubbing together of all surfaces of the hands lathered in soap, followed by rinsing under a stream of water. Hand washing may be accomplished with the use of plain soap, antimicrobial soap, or an antiseptic hand wash and is always indicated when hands are visibly soiled or when performing a surgical scrub. Hand hygiene may involve an alcohol-based hand rub also known as a waterless antiseptic agent. The majority of alcohol-based hand antiseptics contain isopropanol, ethanol, n-propanol, or a combination of two of these products. Alcohol-based hand rubs for HCWs are available as low viscosity rinses, gels, and foams. Alcohol-based hand sanitizers should not be used whenever contamination with spore-producing organisms are suspected, such as *Bacillus anthracis* (see Chapter 17: Bioterrorism) or *Clostridium difficile*.

Despite the well-established benefits of hand hygiene, adherence to this recommended practice remains low. The techniques for hand washing and the use of hand gel are straightforward unless the donning of a surgical gown is involved. Other factors, such as nail hygiene and jewelry, may influence the benefits of hand decontamination. Long fingernails, artificial nails, and chipped nail polish have been associated with high concentrations of microorganisms, which remain present even after careful hand washing or the use of surgical scrubs. Long fingernails and artificial nails have been implicated in the transmission of gram-negative bacilli and yeast. Therefore, fingernails should be kept trim, and nail polish or artificial nails should not be worn. Similarly, the skin underneath rings also has higher concentrations of microorganisms compared with the skin of fingers without rings. However, it is not clear if jewelry results in increased transmission of HAIs.

BASIC INFECTION CONTROL

Technique for Hand Washing

1. Wet hands first with water.
2. Apply an amount of product recommended by the manufacturer to hands.
3. Rub hands together vigorously for at least 15 seconds, covering all surfaces of the hands and fingers (Figure 1.1).
4. Rinse hands with water.
5. Dry thoroughly with a disposable towel.
   a. Wet hands harbor more microorganisms than dry ones.
6. Use towel to turn off the faucet (Figure 1.2).
7. Avoid using hot water because repeated exposure to hot water may increase the risk of dermatitis.
8. Do not touch any part of the sink. If you do, wash again.
9. Lotion or barrier cream can be applied if needed. (Adapted from CDC, 2002)

Technique for Applying Alcohol-Based Hand Rub

1. Apply product to palm of one hand (Figure 1.3). (Follow the manufacturer's recommendations regarding the volume of product to use.)
2. Rub hands together.
3. Ensure that all surfaces of hands and fingers are covered.

FIGURE **1.1**
Technique for hand washing

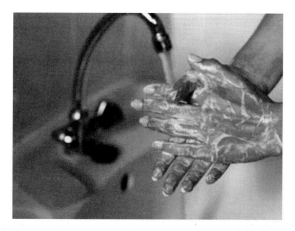

FIGURE **1.2**
Handwashing steps

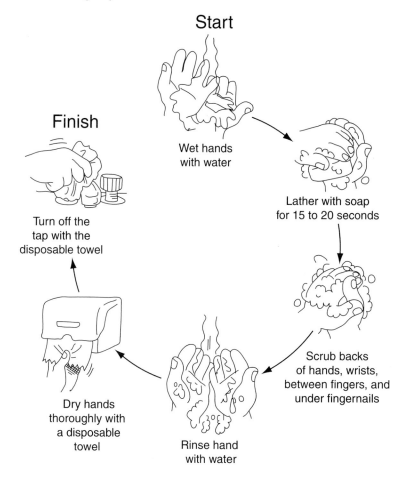

Start

Wet hands
with water

Lather with soap
for 15 to 20 seconds

Scrub backs
of hands, wrists,
between fingers, and
under fingernails

Rinse hand
with water

Dry hands
thoroughly with
a disposable
towel

Turn off the
tap with the
disposable towel

Finish

FIGURE **1.3**

Technique for applying
alcohol-based hand rub

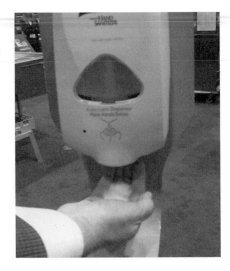

4. Continue rubbing until hands are dry.
5. Lotion or barrier cream can be applied if needed. (Adapted from CDC, 2002)

Technique for Surgical Scrub

1. Remove rings, watches, and bracelets before beginning the surgical hand scrub.
2. Don face mask, surgical shoe covers, and other personal protective equipment (PPE) as required
3. Open brush, and place opened package on sink.
4. Do not touch sink with any part of the body.
5. Wet hands and arms.
6. Surgical prewash:
   a. Apply antiseptic soap, thoroughly lather, and wash the hands and arms to 2 inches above the elbows.
7. Thoroughly rinse hands and arms, keeping hands and wrists higher than the elbows.
8. Brush Method for Scrubbing:
   a. Treat your fingers, hands, and arms as four-sided objects, and scrub each section separately.
   b. Remove debris from underneath fingernails using a nail cleaner under running water.
   c. Pick up the scrub brush.
   d. Wet the scrub brush, and work up a lather.
   e. Scrub hands and forearms for the length of time recommended by the manufacturer, usually 2–6 minutes. (Long scrub times, e.g., 10 minutes, are not necessary.)

   f. Scrub the first hand.

     i. Start at the little finger-side or thumb-side of the hand and scrub the four sides of each digit.

     ii. Scrub the palm, sides of the hand, back of the hand, and the web space between the thumb and index finger.

   g. Scrub your arm in sections of three or four between the wrist and elbow.

   h. Switch hands and repeat.

   i. Thoroughly rinse hands and arms, keeping hands and wrists higher than the elbows.

   j. Dry hands and arms using a sterile towel starting with fingers and hands and ending with arms and elbows. (Adapted from CDC, 2002, and Academy of Health Sciences, Department of Nursing Science, Operating Room Branch)

Technique for Using an Alcohol-Based Surgical Hand Scrub

1. Ensure the product has persistent antimicrobial activity.
2. Follow the manufacturer's directions for use (DFU).
3. Prewash hands and forearms with a non-antimicrobial soap.
4. Thoroughly rinse hands and forearms.
5. Dry hands and forearms completely.
6. Apply the alcohol-based product as recommended.
7. Allow hands and forearms to dry thoroughly before donning sterile gloves.

Observed barriers to hand washing include male sex and physician status, while hand irritation, insufficient time, and lack of resources are among those self-reported barriers. Education and motivation programs for HCWs may be beneficial.

FACTORS INFLUENCING HAND-HYGIENE PRACTICES

The following is adapted from "Improving Compliance With Hand Hygiene in Hospitals," by D. Pittet, 2000. *Infect Control Hosp Epdemiol, 21*, 381–386.

Observed Risk Factors to Poor Adherence to Hand-Hygiene Practices

- Physician rather than nurse
- Nursing assistant rather than nurse
- Male sex
- Working in an intensive-care unit
- Working during the week rather than weekend
- Wearing gowns/gloves
- Automated sink
- Activities with high risk of cross-transmission
- High number of opportunities for hand hygiene per hour of patient care

Self-Reported Factors for Poor Adherence with Hand Hygiene

- Hand-washing agents cause irritation and dryness
- Sinks are inconveniently located or in insufficient number
- Lack of soap and paper towels
- Too busy/insufficient time
- Understaffing/overcrowding
- Patient needs take priority
- Hand hygiene interferes with patient relationship
- Low risk of acquiring infection from patients
- Belief that gloves obviate the need for hand hygiene
- Lack of knowledge of guidelines
- Forgetfulness
- No role model from colleagues or superiors
- Skepticism about the value of hand hygiene
- Disagreement with recommendations

"The CDC recommends that HCWs wear gloves to reduce the risk of personnel acquiring infections from patients, prevent HCW flora from being transmitted to patients, and reduce transient contamination of HCW hands by flora that can be transmitted from one patient to another" (CDC, 2002). When sterile gloves are needed, without the need for a sterile gown, the open gloving technique is used. In other situations, sterile gloves and gown are necessary. In this case, the sterile technique for gowning and closed gloving should be followed to prevent contamination and infection.

Technique for Open Gloving

1. Remove all jewelry from hands.
2. Perform appropriate hand hygiene.
3. Peel apart outer glove wrapping, and carefully remove inner package.
4. Place inner package on a clean, flat surface.
5. Open package without touching gloves.
6. Grasp the cuff edge with the thumb and first two fingers of one hand (Figure 1.4).
7. Line up the thumb side of the glove with the thumb side of the other hand.
8. Touch only the glove's inside surface.
9. Slip the glove over the fingers and thumb.
10. Ensure that the cuff edge does not fold over.
11. With the gloved hand, slip the first two fingers underneath second glove's cuff.
12. Slip second glove over the ungloved hand.
13. Ensure that the gloved hand does not touch any exposed skin.
14. Adjust the gloves to ensure a tight fit over the fingers and thumb.

Doffing Gloves

15. Grasp one glove at the wrist/cuff level without touching exposed skin.
16. Remove glove, turning it inside out, then discard.

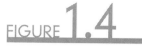

FIGURE 1.4

Open gloving

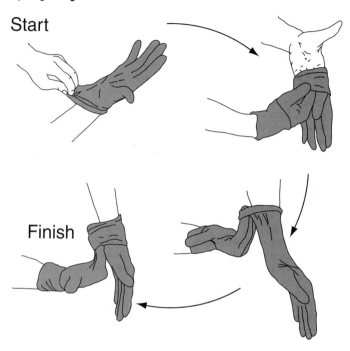

17. Take first two fingers of bare hand and tuck inside the remaining glove without touching outside of glove.
18. Remove glove, turning it inside out, then discard.

Technique for Gowning and Closed Gloving

The following is adapted from Academy of Health Sciences, Department of Nursing Science, Operating Room Branch.

Gowning

1. Remove rings, watches, and bracelets before beginning the surgical hand scrub.
2. Don face mask, surgical shoe covers, and other personal protective equipment (PPE) as required (Figure 1.5).
3. Perform appropriate hand hygiene.
4. Circulating nurse opens sterile gown and glove packages.
5. Grasp the gown from the inside of the neck and lift it from the sterile field.
6. Step back and allow the gown to unfold without touching the sterile field.

FIGURE 1.5

Gowning

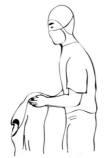

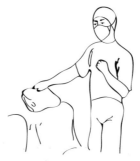

1. Perform appropriate hand hygiene and dry hands

2. Pick up gown from inside of the neck and lift it from the sterile field

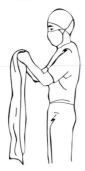

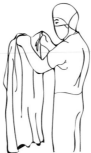

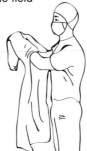

3. Let gown unfold

4. Open the gown to locate sleeve/armholes

5. Slip arms into sleeves

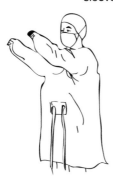

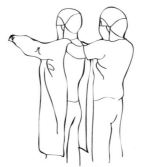

6. Hold arms out and slightly up

7. Circulating nurse pulls the gown on and secures it

7. Locate the arm holes and gently insert both hands into the gown simultaneously, leaving your hands within the sleeves.
8. The circulating nurse brings the gown over the shoulders and secures the back of the gown.

9. Have circulating nurse securely tie back of gown at neck and waist. (If gown is a wrap-around style, sterile flap to cover gown is not touched until the nurse has gloved.)

Closed Gloving

10. With hands covered by gown sleeves, open the sterile glove package.
11. Pinch the bottom of the glove through the gown, and lift it out of the package.
12. With palm up, place the palm of the glove over the gowned hand.
13. The fingers of the glove will point toward your elbow.
14. Grasp the glove by the cuff using the other gowned hand, and stretch the glove over the gown cuff while working your fingers out of the gown cuff and into the glove.
15. Unroll the glove cuff so that it covers the stockinette sleeve cuff.
16. Never touch the outside of the gown with the bare hands.
17. Repeat steps 11 through 16 and glove the other hand.
18. Adjust the gloves to ensure a tight fit over the fingers and thumb.

Tying the Gown

19. Grasp the top portion of the cardboard tab of the waist tie, and hand it to the circulating nurse.
20. Turn and grasp the waist tie, and secure it to the front of the gown.

INFECTION PRECAUTIONS

In addition to hand hygiene, standard precautions and transmission-based precautions are used in infection control and prevention. Standard precautions are intended to be applied to the care of all patients in all health care settings, even if the HCW comes in contact with blood, body fluids, secretions, and excretions regardless of the suspected or confirmed presence of an infectious agent (Brevis Corporation, 2007). Standard precautions include the use of hand hygiene, PPE, and respiratory hygiene. Standard precautions help to reduce the risk of transmission of microorganisms from recognized and unrecognized sources of infection in hospitals. Standard precautions are applied to all patients regardless of diagnosis or infection status. The CDC's standard precautions incorporate all requirements of the Occupational Safety & Health Administration (OSHA) bloodborne pathogens standard. Transmission-based precautions are designed for patients suspected of or documented with highly transmissible or epidemiologically important pathogens for which additional precautions beyond standard precautions are needed. The three types of transmission-based precautions are airborne precautions, droplet precautions, and contact precautions.

Droplet Precautions

Droplet precautions are recommended for patients known or suspected to be infected with pathogens transmitted by respiratory droplets that are generated by a patient who is coughing, sneezing, or talking. Respiratory droplets carrying infectious organisms travel directly from the infected person to the mucosal surfaces of the recipient generally over short distances. The maximum distance for droplet transmission is currently unresolved but had been agreed to be a distance of 3 feet or less around the patient. However, more recent studies suggest transmission may occur with distances between 6 and 10 feet. Droplet size, another area for consideration, has traditionally been defined as having particles that are larger than 5 micrometers in size (Siegel, Rhinehart, Jackson, Chiarello, & the Healthcare Infection Control Practices Advisory Committee [HICPAC]). In an acute care facility, these patients should be placed in a single room. Anyone who enters the room should wear a mask. However, eye protection is not necessary. These patients should only be transported outside of their rooms when medically necessary (Brevis Corporation, 2007).

Airborne Precautions

Airborne precautions are recommended for patients known or suspected to be infected with infectious agents transmitted person-to-person by the airborne route. This occurs when droplet particles that are small in size, usually smaller than 5 micrometers in diameter, remain suspended in air and are therefore able to travel over longer distances. As such, face-to-face contact is not necessary for infectious transmission. Given the small size of the droplet particles, a surgical mask is insufficient protection in these cases (Siegel et al., 2007). For example, patients with *Mycobacterium tuberculosis* or chicken pox should be subject to airborne precautions. These include placement in an isolation room, use of fit-tested National Institute for Occupational Safety and Health (NIOSH)-approved N95 or higher respirators (disposable particulate respirators that filter at least 95% of airborne particles but is not resistant to oil) and the limitation of patient transport outside of the patient's room (Brevis Corporation, 2007).

Contact Precautions

Contact precautions are recommended for patients with known or suspected infections or evidence of syndromes that represent an increased risk for contact transmission. In this type of precaution, gloves and gowns should be worn upon entry into the patient's room. Disposable noncritical patient-care equipment or the use of patient-dedicated equipment should be used, when possible (Brevis Corporation, 2007).

IMMUNOCOMPROMISED PATIENTS

Immunocompromised patients vary in their susceptibility to nosocomial infections, depending on the severity and duration of immunosuppression. They generally are at increased risk for bacterial, fungal, parasitic, and viral infections from both endogenous and exogenous sources. The use of standard precautions for all patients and transmission-based precautions for specified patients, as recommended in this guideline, should reduce the acquisition by these patients of institutionally acquired bacteria from other patients and environments.

It is beyond the scope of this guideline to address the various measures that may be used for immunocompromised patients to delay or prevent acquisition of potential pathogens during temporary periods of neutropenia. Rather, the primary objective of this guideline is to prevent transmission of pathogens from infected or colonized patients in hospitals.

POST-TEST QUESTIONS

1-1. Appropriate hand hygiene can:
   a. Increase the risk of mortality
   b. Increase the rate of nosocomial infections
   c. Prevent the transmission of microorganisms
   d. Increase costs of health care–associated infections
1-2. Hands must be washed with soap and water:
   a. When the hands are visibly dirty
   b. After contact with a patient's intact skin
   c. Before caring for patients with severe neutropenia or other forms of severe immunosuppression
   d. After removing gloves
1-3. Which of the following is TRUE regarding hand washing?
   a. The water should be hot.
   b. Hands and forearm should be kept higher than elbows during washing.
   c. Hands should be washed for a minimum of 60 seconds.
   d. Hands should be dried thoroughly from fingers to wrists and forearms with paper towel, single-use cloth, or warm air dryer.
1-4. Which of the following is TRUE regarding the use of alcohol-based hand gels?
   a. Apply an ample amount of product to completely cover both hands.
   b. Rub hands together, covering all surfaces of hands and fingers with antiseptic.
   c. Rub hands together for several minutes until alcohol is dry.
   d. If gloves are to be used, put gloves on while hands are still wet from the gel.
1-5. Which of the following infectious precautions should be applied to a foreign-born national who is currently incarcerated and is being evaluated in the emergency department for fever, weight loss, pleuritic chest pain, and cough productive of bloody secretions of more than 3 weeks duration?
   a. Standard precautions
   b. Contact precautions
   c. Droplet precautions
   d. Airborne precautions

References

Academy of Health Sciences, Department of Nursing Science, Operating Room Branch. (n.d.). *Scrub, gown, and glove techniques*. Retrieved February 22, 2010, from: http://www.dns.amedd. army.mil/91d/Rapidtrainup/CD1/SMScrbGwnGlv.doc

Brevis Corporation. http://www.brevis.com

Centers for Disease Control and Prevention (CDC). (2002). Guideline for hand hygiene in health-care settings: Recommendations of the Healthcare Infection Control Practices Advisory Committee and the HICPAC/SHEA/APIC/IDSA Hand Hygiene Task Force. *Morbidity and Mortality Weekly Report, 51*(RR16).

Pittet, D. (2000). Improving compliance with hand hygiene in hospitals. *Infection Control and Hospital Epidemiology, 21,* 381–386.

Siegel, J.D., Rhinehart, E., Jackson, M., Chiarello, L., & the Healthcare Infection Control Practices Advisory Committee (HICPAC). (2007). 2007 Guideline for isolation precautions: Preventing transmission of infectious agents in healthcare settings. Retrieved July 14, 2010, from http://www.cdc.gov/ncidod/dhqp/pdf/isolation2007.pdf

Web Sites

http://eclipse.cps.k12.va.us/Schools/DCC/nurse3.html
http://www.handwashingforlife.com/files/images/2-apply-purell.jpg
http://tpub.com/content/medical/14295/css/14295_109.htm
http://utmb.edu/surgery/clerks/glove1.jpg
http://wiki.unt.edu/display/RMS/Radiation+Safety+Committee

Bloodborne Pathogen Standard

2

This chapter includes topics on bloodborne pathogens and exposure-control plans and discusses the methods of transmission of bloodborne pathogens. Also, the use of personal protective equipment is reviewed. There is discussion differentiating between the Exposure Control Plan and the Post-Exposure Control Plan. HIV, hepatitis B, and hepatitis C are discussed. The Occupational Safety and Health Administration (OSHA)–issued Bloodborne Pathogens Standard (29 CFR 1910.1030) is discussed. Splash exposures and needlestick injuries are described.

OBJECTIVES

1. Identify bloodborne pathogens.
2. Define the OSHA Bloodborne Pathogen Standard.
3. Explain the methods of transmission of bloodborne pathogens.
4. Discuss the appropriate use of personal protective equipment (PPE).
5. Differentiate between the Exposure Control Plan and the Post-Exposure Control Plan.

PRE-TEST QUESTIONS

2-1. Health care facilities are required to have the following policies and procedures in place to protect the health care worker from exposure to bloodborne pathogens:
a. Exposure Control Plan
b. Post-Exposure Control Plan
c. Both a and b
d. Only a

2-2. Which of the following are not considered bloodborne pathogens:
   a. Hepatitis B
   b. Hepatitis C
   c. HIV
   d. Tuberculosis
2-3. As a health care worker, you should be immunized against:
   a. Hepatitis B
   b. Hepatitis C
   c. HIV
   d. Hepatitis B and hepatitis C
2-4. Once you have been immunized against hepatitis B, with the series of three injections at now, at 1 month, and at 6 months, you:
   a. Have a lifetime immunity
   b. Should have a titer drawn to evaluate immunity post-series
   c. Should repeat the series every 10 years
   d. None of the above
2-5. Examples of engineering controls that eliminate or reduce the risk of bloodborne pathogen transmission include all of the following except:
   a. Hand-wash facilities
   b. Sharps containers
   c. Needleless delivery systems
   d. Use of high efficiency particulate air (HEPA) filtrations

Workers in many different occupations are at risk of exposure to bloodborne pathogens, including hepatitis B, hepatitis C, and HIV/AIDS. First-aid team members, housekeeping personnel in some settings, nurses, and other health care providers are examples of workers who may be at risk of exposure.

In 1991 OSHA issued the Bloodborne Pathogens Standard (29 CFR 1910.1030) to protect workers from this risk. In 2001, in response to the Needlestick Safety and Prevention Act, OSHA revised the Bloodborne Pathogens Standard. The revised standard clarifies the need for employers to select safer needle devices and to involve employees in identifying and choosing these devices. The updated standard also requires employers to maintain a log of injuries from contaminated sharps (OSHA Log 300, 2004).

HIV/AIDS

HIV is transmitted by contact with infected body fluids, including blood, semen, vaginal secretions, and breast milk. Transmission of HIV occurs through sexual intercourse with an infected partner, exposure to HIV-infected blood, blood products or HIV-contaminated equipment, and perinatal transmission during pregnancy, at the time of delivery, or through breastfeeding (World Health Organization [WHO], 2005). HIV-infected individuals can transmit HIV to others within a few days after becoming infected and then indefinitely.

HEPATITIS B VIRUS

Hepatitis B is a serious liver infection caused by the hepatitis B virus (HBV). HBV infection can cause acute illness and lead to chronic or lifelong infection, cirrhosis of the liver, liver cancer, liver failure, and death. HBV is transmitted through percutaneous or mucosal contact with infectious blood or body fluids. Hepatitis B vaccination is the most effective measure to prevent HBV infection and its consequences and is recommended for all infants and others at risk for HBV infection (Centers for Disease Control and Prevention, 2005, 2006). (See Chapter 3, "Immunizations.")

HEPATITIS C VIRUS

Hepatitis C is a liver disease caused by the hepatitis C virus (HCV) that sometimes results in an acute illness but most often becomes a silent, chronic infection that can lead to cirrhosis, liver failure, liver cancer, and death. Chronic HCV infection develops in a majority of HCV-infected persons, most of whom do not know they are infected because they have no symptoms. HCV is spread by contact with blood or body fluids of an infected person. There is no vaccine for hepatitis C.

Employers are required to protect employees from occupational hazards. One example of an occupational hazard is health care worker (HCW) and emergency medical personnel exposure to blood and other potentially infectious materials (OPIM). Puncture wounds are the most common means of work-related transmission. The risk of infection after a needlestick exposure in HIV-infected blood is 0.3%–0.4% (or 3–4 out of 1,000). The risk is higher if the exposure involves blood from a patient with a high viral load, a deep puncture wound, a needle with a hollow bore and visible blood, a device used for venous or arterial access, or a patient who dies within 60 days after the needlestick injury to the HCW.

Splash exposures of blood on skin with an open lesion present some risk, but it is much lower than from a puncture wound (CDC, 2001). An exposure can also be the result of a splash of blood or OPIM into the mouth or eyes. The employee should be instructed, during orientation, as to the locations of eye wash stations in the event of an accidental splash. In the event of an exposure, the employee should immediately ask for assistance and go to the eye wash station, let the water run for a few seconds to rid the system of old water or other elements, then keep the face and eyes under the flowing water for approximately 10 minutes based on the institution's policy. The employee should then follow institution policy regarding subsequent care (e.g., report to employee health or to the hospital emergency department for follow-up).

Employers must have a plan in place to protect HCWs from occupational exposure to blood and bloodborne pathogens. In the event of such an exposure, post-exposure prophylaxis (PEP) must be discussed with the employee.

If an employee has an exposure to bloodborne pathogens that is a result of a needlestick injury or a splash, the employee must immediately report the exposure to his or her supervisor (Figure 2.1). The employee must be triaged,

FIGURE **2.1**

Employee with needle stick injury

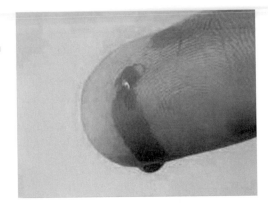

Courtesy of www.wormsandgermsblog.com

counseled, and offered post-exposure medication within two hours of the exposure incident and undergo blood work for baseline studies. Depending on policy, the employee will be tested for hepatitis B, hepatitis C, and HIV. The blood tests are typically repeated, according to policy, but usually at 6 weeks, 3 months, and then again at 6 months post-exposure. All individuals who undergo HIV testing must receive pre- and post-test counseling. The physician of the patient who was involved in the employee exposure will be notified of the exposure and will ask the patient if he or she is also willing to undergo blood testing because the employee had an exposure. If the patient agrees to be tested, the employee has the right to know the results of the patient's blood work, which may influence both the employee's decision to take prophylactic medications and the duration of medication therapy. The post-exposure report typically contains the patient's significant medical history to determine the risk of disease transmission, such as a history of multiple blood transfusions, HIV status, hepatitis B and C status, and history of intravenous drug use. The patient history, the level of exposure—superficial needlestick, deep-tissue penetration with blood injection, mucus membrane splash, and so on—and the side-effect profile are included as part of counseling and are factors that may affect the employee's decision to initiate prophylactic medication.

PRE- AND POST-TEST COUNSELING ASSOCIATED WITH HIV-ANTIBODY TESTING

General Guidelines

People who are being tested for HIV are frequently fearful about the test results.

- Establish rapport with the patient.
- Assess the patient's ability to understand HIV counseling.
- Determine the patient's ability to access support systems.
- Educate the patient on methods to reduce the risk of future exposures.
- Refer the patient to early intervention and support programs.

▇ Be aware of confidentiality issues. Breaches of confidentiality have led to discrimination. A positive test result affects all aspects of the patient's life (personal, social, economic, etc.) and can raise difficult emotions (anger, anxiety, guilt, and thoughts of suicide).

Pre-Test Counseling

1. Determine the patient's risk factors and when the last risk occurred. Counseling should be individualized according to these parameters.
2. Provide education to decrease future risk of exposure.
3. Provide education that will help the patient protect sexual and drug-sharing partners.
4. Discuss problems related to the delay between infection and an accurate test result. Testing will need to be repeated at intervals for up to 6 months after each possible exposure. Discuss the need to use measures to decrease the risks to the patient and the patient's partners during that interval.
5. Discuss the possibility of false-negative tests, which are most likely to occur during the window period.
6. Assess support systems. Provide telephone numbers and resources as needed.
7. Discuss the patient's personally anticipated responses to test results (both positive and negative).
8. Outline assistance that will be offered if the test is positive.

Post-Test Counseling

1. If the test is negative, reinforce pre-test counseling and prevention education. Remind the patient that the test needs to be repeated at intervals for up to 6 months after the most recent exposure risk.
2. If the test is positive, understand that the patient may be in shock and may not hear much of what you say.
3. Provide resources for medical and emotional support and help the patient get immediate assistance.
   - Evaluate suicide risk and follow-up as needed.
   - Determine the need to test others who have had high-risk contact with the patient.
   - Discuss retesting to verify results. This tactic supports hope for the patient, but more importantly, it keeps the patient in the system. While waiting for the second test result, the patient has time to think about and adjust to the possibility of being HIV-infected.
   - Encourage optimism.
4. Remind the patient that effective treatments are available; HIV is not a death sentence.
5. Review health habits that can improve the immune system.
6. Arrange for the patient to speak to HIV-infected people who are willing to share with and assist newly diagnosed patients during the transition period.

7. Reinforce that a positive HIV test means that the patient is infected, but does not necessarily mean that the patient has progressed to AIDS.

8. Educate to prevent new infections. HIV-infected people should be instructed to avoid donating blood, organs, or semen; to avoid sharing razors, toothbrushes, or other household items that may contain blood or other body fluids; and to protect sexual and needle-sharing partners from blood, semen, and vaginal secretions (Lewis, Heitkemper, Dirksen, O'Brien, & Bucher, 2007).

EXPOSURE CONTROL PLAN

Health care facilities are required to have an Exposure Control Plan in place. This plan is in place to eliminate or minimize employee exposure to blood or OPIM through compliance with the OSHA Bloodborne Pathogens Standard. The plan includes methods such as standard precautions (see Chapter 1, "Basic Infection Control"), engineering and work practice controls, PPE, housekeeping control, hepatitis B vaccination, communication of hazards to employees and training (see Chapter 12, "Spills"), proper record keeping, and procedures for evaluating the circumstances surrounding an exposure incident.

Engineering and Work Practice Controls

Engineering and work practice controls must be used to eliminate or reduce employee exposure and must be reviewed on a regular basis to ensure effectiveness. These include: (a) hand-washing facilities, (b) the use of safety needles, (Figures 2.2–2.6) (c) needleless systems for medication delivery (Figure 2.7),

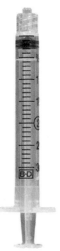

FIGURE 2.2

Luer-Lok Syringe

Courtesy and © Becton, Dickinson and Company.

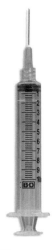

FIGURE 2.3

**BD 10 mL Syringe/
Needle Combination
BD Luer-Lok Tip**

Courtesy and © Becton, Dickinson and Company.

FIGURE 2.4

Safety needle

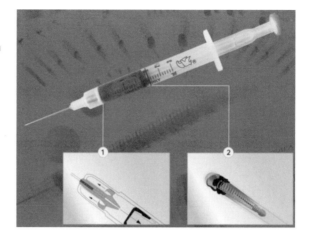

FIGURE 2.5

Safety glide needle before activation

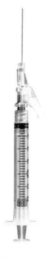

Courtesy and © Becton, Dickinson and Company.

FIGURE 2.6

Safety glide needle after activation

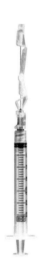

Courtesy and © Becton, Dickinson and Company.

(d) sufficient numbers and appropriate placement of sharps containers, (e) appropriate handling of medical waste (see Chapter 11, "Medical Waste Disposal"), and (f) appropriate handling of laundry services, if applicable.

Hepatitis B Vaccination

Employees such as HCWs and emergency medical personnel are at the highest risk for occupational exposure to infectious diseases. Their employers must offer

FIGURE **2.7**

Needles IV system

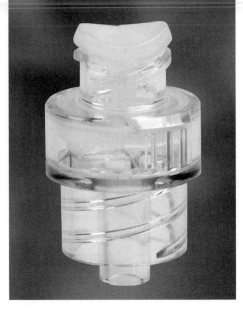

Courtesy and © Becton, Dickinson and Company.

them hepatitis B vaccination at no cost (Figure 2.8). Vaccination is encouraged unless: (a) documentation exists that the employee has previously received the series, (b) antibody testing indicates that the employee is immune, or (c) medical evaluation shows that vaccination is contraindicated. Employees must sign an acceptance/declination form.

Should an employee at risk for hepatitis B choose to decline vaccination, the employee must sign a declination form. Employees who decline may request and obtain the vaccination at a later date at no cost. Documentation of refusal of the vaccination is kept on file.

Personal Protective Equipment

OSHA also mandates that employers must provide, make accessible, and require the use of PPE at no cost to the employee. PPE must also be provided in appropriate sizes. Hypoallergenic gloves or other similar alternatives must be made available to employees who have allergic sensitivities to gloves and glove components such as latex and glove powder (see Table 2.1).

FIGURE 2.8

Hepatitis B injection administration

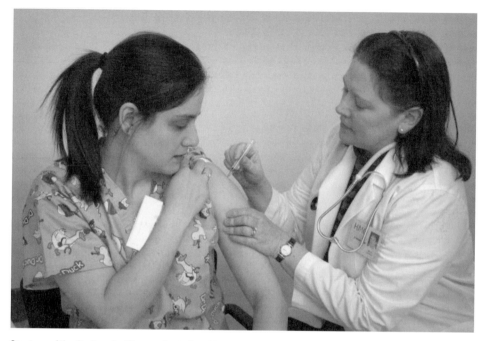

Courtesy of the Centers for Disease Control and Prevention/Judy Schmidt. Photo by James Gathany.

TABLE 2.1

OSHA Requirements for PPE to Minimize Exposure to Bloodborne Pathogens

EQUIPMENT	INDICATIONS FOR USE
Gloves	Must be used when it can be reasonably anticipated that the employee may have contact with blood or other potentially infectious materials, when performing vascular access procedures, and when handling or touching contaminated items or surfaces. Gloves must be replaced if torn, punctured, or contaminated or if their ability to function as a barrier is compromised.

(Continued)

TABLE **2.1**

(*Continued*)

EQUIPMENT	INDICATIONS FOR USE
Clothing (gowns, aprons, caps, boots)	Must be used when occupational exposure is anticipated. The type and characteristics will depend on the task and degree of exposure anticipated.
Facial protection (mask with glasses with solid side shields or a chin-length face shield)	Must be used when splashes, sprays, spatters, or droplets of blood or other potentially infectious materials pose a hazard to the eyes, nose, or mouth.

From: OSHA.

POST-TEST QUESTIONS

2-1. Health care facilities are required to have the following policies and procedures in place to protect the health care worker from exposure to bloodborne pathogens:
 a. Exposure Control Plan
 b. Post-Exposure Control Plan
 c. Both a and b
 d. Only a

2-2. Which of the following are not considered bloodborne pathogens:
 a. Hepatitis B
 b. Hepatitis C
 c. HIV
 d. Tuberculosis

2-3. As a health care worker, you should be immunized against:
 a. Hepatitis B
 b. Hepatitis C
 c. HIV
 d. Hepatitis B and hepatitis C

2-4. Once you have been immunized against hepatitis B, with the series of three injections now, at 1 month, and at 6 months, you:
 a. Have a lifetime immunity
 b. Should have a titer drawn to evaluate immunity post-series
 c. Should repeat the series every 10 years
 d. None of the above

2-5. Examples of engineering controls that eliminate or reduce the risk of bloodborne pathogen transmission include all of the following except:
 a. Hand-wash facilities
 b. Sharps containers
 c. Needleless delivery systems
 d. Use of HEPA filtrations

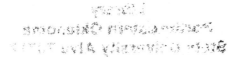

References

Centers for Disease Control and Prevention. (1998). Public Health Service guidelines for the management of health-care worker exposures to HIV and recommendations for postexposure prophylaxis. *MMWR, 47*(RR-7), 1–28.

Centers for Disease Control and Prevention. (2001). Updated U.S. Public Health Service guidelines for the management of occupational exposures to HBV, HCV, and HIV and recommendations for postexposure prophylaxis. *MMWR, 50*(RR11), 1–42.

Centers for Disease Control and Prevention. (2005). A comprehensive immunization strategy to eliminate transmission of hepatitis B virus infection in the United States. Part I: Immunization of infants, children and adolescents. *MMWR, 54*(RR-16), 1–39.

Centers for Disease Control and Prevention. (2006). A comprehensive immunization strategy to eliminate transmission of hepatitis B virus infection in the United States. Part II: Immunization of adults. *MMWR, 55*(RR-16), 1–25.

Lewis, S., Heitkemper, M., Dirksen, S., O'Brien, P., & Bucher, L. (2007). *Medical-surgical nursing* (7th ed.). St. Louis, MO: Mosby Elsevier.

OSHA bloodborne pathogen standard. Retrieved October 16, 2008, from http://www.osha.gov/SLTC/bloodbornepathogens/

World Health Organization (WHO). (2005, June 29). Access to HIV treatment continues to accelerated in developing countries, but bottlenecks persist says WHO. UNAIDS Report, Press Release. Retrieved April 22, 2006, from http://www.who.int/3by5/progressreportJune2005/en/

Web Sites

http://www.bd.com/medical-surgical/pdfs/BD_Medical_Catalog.pdf

http://www.bd.com/us/diabetes/hcp/main.aspx?cat=3067&id=3127

http://catalog.bd.com/bdCat/attributeSearch.doCustomer?priority=0&categoryID=R142

http://www.ccsyringe.com/images/safety-syringe.jpg

http://www.cdc.gov/about/organization/mission.htm

http://www.cdcnpin.org/scripts/hepatitis/index.asp#overview

http://www.gsk.com.hk/ProductPopUp.aspx?ID=163&ProductType=vaccines

http://www.osha.gov/

http://www.osha.gov/as/opa/missionposter.html

http://www.osha.gov/SLTC/bloodbornepathogens/

www.osha.gov/SLTC/bloodbornepathogens/

http://www.stdmed.net/images/img_pharm037.jpg

http://www.wormsandgermsblog.com/tags/needlestick-injuries/

Immunizations

3

This chapter includes topics on standard immunizations for the pediatric and adult populations. The three methods of vaccine administration are reviewed. The content differentiates between live and attenuated vaccines. There is discussion on the American Academy of Pediatrics recommendations. The content topics include discussion of the following vaccines: inactivated diphtheria, tetanus, and pertussis (DPT); live attenuated, tetanus; Td, a tetanus-diphtheria vaccine; Haemophilus influenza type b (Hib); hepatitis A; hepatitis B; herpes zoster; H1N1; human papillomavirus (HPV); influenza; meningococcal; measles, mumps, and rubella; pneumococcal; poliomyelitis; rotavirus; and varicella. Finally, vaccine safety and common risks associated with immunizations are discussed.

OBJECTIVES

1. Identify standard immunizations for the pediatric and adult populations.
2. Define immunization.
3. Explain three methods of vaccine administration.
4. Discuss the most common risks associated with immunizations.
5. Differentiate between live and attenuated vaccines.

PRE-TEST QUESTIONS

3-1. Which of the following vaccines is considered a live vaccine?
    a. Hemophilus influenza
    b. Hepatitis B
    c. Pneumococcal
    d. Varicella
3-2. Live vaccines may be contraindicated in patients with:
    a. Immunosuppression
    b. Growth hormone deficiency
    c. Allergy to thimerosal

       d. A previous reaction to pertussis vaccine

3-3. Which of the following is not a route of administration for common vaccines?
    a. Subcutaneous
    b. Intramuscular
    c. Oral
    d. Intravenous

3-4. Which of the following populations is at high risk of being exposed to the hepatitis B virus and therefore should be immunized?
    a. College freshmen living in dormitories
    b. U.S. military recruits
    c. Health care workers
    d. Adults ages 19–64 who have asthma

3-5. Which of the following vaccines is designed to prevent shingles?
    a. Pneumococcal vaccine
    b. Hepatitis A vaccine
    c. Human papillomavirus vaccine
    d. Herpes zoster vaccine

Immunization is the process where a person is made immune or resistant to an infectious disease, usually by the administration of a vaccine. Vaccines stimulate the body to protect against subsequent infection. Immunization is a proven tool for improving quality of life by controlling and eliminating life-threatening infectious diseases and is estimated to avert more than 2 million deaths each year. It is one of the most cost-effective health care–related investments. Societal benefits include creation and maintenance of herd immunity against communicable diseases, prevention of disease outbreaks, and reduction in health care–related costs (Centers for Disease Control and Prevention, 2006; World Health Organization, 2010).

An immunization schedule in the United States for children and adults is approved by the Advisory Committee on Immunization Practices (ACIP), the American Academy of Pediatrics (AAP), and the American Academy of Family Physicians (AAFP). Information about the recommended schedule for routine administration of vaccines to healthy children, adolescents, and adults; a catch-up schedule for children aged 4 months to 6 years; and a catch-up schedule for children ages 7 to 18 years are provided and updated annually.

INACTIVATED AND LIVE ATTENUATED VACCINES

There are two types of vaccines: inactivated vaccines and live attenuated vaccines. *Inactivated vaccines* can be made of either whole bacteria or viruses or parts of these organisms. These vaccines are not alive and cannot replicate in the body. Examples of inactivated vaccines include hepatitis A and B, influenza injection, pneumococcal, and meningococcal. In general, inactivated vaccines require three to five doses to provide optimal immunity, and antibody titers wane over time. Conversely, live attenuated vaccines are a weakened form of the virus or bacteria and must replicate within the body in order to be effective. The immune response by the body simulates the response seen after acquiring the actual disease. Examples of live attenuated vaccines include varicella, rotavirus, and intranasal influenza vaccines. These vaccines may be contraindicated in patients who are immunocompromised or in those patients who live with someone that is immunocompromised because of the possibility of transmitting the actual disease to a person with a weakened immune system.

Diphtheria, Tetanus, and Pertussis Vaccines (DPT)

Diphtheria is caused by a bacterium, *Corynebacterium diphtheriae*. The disease occurs when the bacteria release a toxin, or poison, into the person's body. Diphtheria bacteria live in the mouth, throat, and nose of an infected person and can be passed to others by droplet transmission such as coughing or sneezing. Occasionally, contact transmission may occur from skin sores or through articles soiled with discharge from sores of infected persons. The initial signs and symptoms of diphtheria infection may be confused with the common cold, in which patients may experience sore throat, mild fever, and chills. But, as the disease progresses, it causes a thick coating at the back of the throat, which can make it difficult to breathe or swallow. Up to 5% to 10% of all people infected with diphtheria die; however, this rate is higher in certain groups such as children younger than 5 years of age and adults older than age 40 years. The most common complications are inflammation of the heart, leading to abnormal heart rhythms, and inflammation of the nerves, which may cause temporary paralysis of some muscles. If the paralysis affects the diaphragm (the major muscle for breathing), the patient may develop pneumonia or respiratory failure.

Tetanus is caused by a toxin made by the spore-forming bacterium *Clostridium tetani*. These spores are difficult to kill because they are not effected by heat or chemicals and are commonly found in the soil, as well as the intestines and feces of humans and many household and farm animals. The bacteria usually enter the human body through a puncture wound. Unlike many other diseases, tetanus is not spread from person to person. The symptoms of tetanus are caused by the tetanus toxin acting on the central nervous system. Usually, the first sign is lockjaw or spasm of the jaw muscles, followed by stiffness of the neck, difficulty in swallowing, and stiffness of the abdominal muscles. Other signs can include fever, sweating, elevated blood pressure, and rapid heart rate. Complete recovery, if it occurs, can take months. Many people infected with tetanus die. Overall, the mortality rate is about 11%, but it can be as high as 18% in persons age 60 years and older and 22% in unvaccinated persons. Laryngospasm or spasm of the vocal cords, bone fractures, and convulsions can complicate the tetanus infection. Other possible complications include hypertension and abnormal heart rhythms.

Pertussis is caused by a bacterium, *Bordetella pertussis*. Pertussis is spread through the air by infectious droplets and is very contagious. Pertussis symptoms are divided into three stages: the catarrhal, paroxysmal, and convalescent stages. In the catarrhal stage, patients experience runny nose, sneezing, low-grade fever, and a mild cough. This stage typically continues for 1 to 2 weeks. Following the catarrhal phase, patients experience the paroxysmal stage, which typically lasts from 1 to 6 weeks but can continue for up to 10 weeks. Symptoms of this phase include frequent bursts of rapid coughs. At the end of each burst or paroxysm the patient makes a high-pitched "whooping cough" due to a long inhalation. Sometimes, infants and young children turn blue and vomit after the coughing burst. The last phase of the disease is the convalescent stage. This typically lasts for 2 to 6 weeks but may last for months. During this stage, the cough usually disappears, but coughing bursts can recur whenever the patient suffers another respiratory infection. Infants and children are most severely affected by pertussis, and deaths can occur in this patient population. In adolescents and adults the disease is usually milder, and the only symptom may be a persistent cough. However, these patients may transmit the disease to others, including unimmunized or incompletely immunized infants. The most common complication associated with pertussis infections is secondary bacterial infection, usually pneumonia. Infants can also develop neurologic complications such as seizures and encephalopathy, most likely because of lack of oxygen to the brain during the coughing bursts.

Vaccination is effective in the prevention of disease caused by diphtheria, tetanus, and pertussis. There are four combination vaccines used to prevent diphtheria, tetanus, and pertussis: DTaP, Tdap, DT, and Td. Two of these (DTaP and DT) are given to children younger than 7 years of age, and two (Tdap and Td) are given to older children and adults.

Upper-case letters in these vaccine abbreviations denote full-strength doses of diphtheria (D) and tetanus (T) toxoids and pertussis (P) vaccine. Lower-case "d" and "p" denote reduced doses of diphtheria and pertussis used in the adolescent/adult-formulations. The "a" in DTaP and Tdap stands for "acellular," meaning that the pertussis component contains only a part of the pertussis organism.

Children should get a total of five doses of DTaP, one dose at each of the following ages: 2 months, 4 months, 6 months, 15–18 months, and 4–6 years. DT does not contain pertussis, and it is used as a substitute for DTaP for children who cannot tolerate the pertussis vaccine (CDC, 2007).

Td is a tetanus-diphtheria vaccine given to adolescents and adults as a booster shot every 10 years, or after an exposure to tetanus under some circumstances. Tdap is similar to Td, but it also contains protection against pertussis. A single dose of Tdap is recommended for adolescents 11 or 12 years of age, or in place of one Td booster in older adolescents and adults age 19 through 64 (CDC, 2007).

Haemophilus Influenza Type B Vaccine (Hib)

The bacterium *Haemophilus influenzae* type b is the cause of Hib disease. There are six different types of these bacteria (a through f). Type b organisms account for almost all of the cases of the invasive disease. Hib disease is spread person-to-person by direct contact or through respiratory droplets. Usually the organisms remain in the nose and throat, but occasionally the bacteria spread to the lungs or bloodstream and cause a serious infection. Symptoms of the disease vary depending on the part of the body infected. The most common type of invasive Hib disease is meningitis. Symptoms of Hib meningitis include fever, decreased mental status, and stiff neck. Patients who survive Hib meningitis infection often suffer some permanent neurologic damage, including blindness, deafness, and mental retardation. Another common Hib infection is epiglottitis, a life-threatening infection and swelling in the throat. Other forms of invasive Hib disease include joint infection, skin infection, pneumonia, and bone infection (CDC, 1998a).

Vaccination with the Hib vaccine has been shown to dramatically reduce the number of Hib infections. Children receive four doses of the Hib vaccine at 2 months of age, 4 months of age, 6 months of age, and 12–15 months of age. Although children older than 5 years usually do not need the Hib vaccine some older children or adults with preexisting medical conditions may benefit from Hib vaccination. These conditions include sickle cell disease, HIV/AIDS, removal of the spleen, bone marrow transplant, or cancer treatment with drugs (CDC, 1998a).

Hepatitis A Vaccine

Hepatitis A is a liver disease caused by hepatitis A virus (HAV). HAV is spread from person to person by fecal–oral route, for example, when an infected person who prepares or handles food doesn't wash their hands adequately after using the toilet and then touches other people's food. In addition, contaminated food, water, and ice can lead to HAV infection in travelers in many areas of the world where HAV is common. Another method of transmission of HAV is during contact with a household member or a sex partner who has hepatitis A. The most common initial symptoms of hepatitis A are the sudden onset of fever, fatigue, anorexia, nausea, abdominal pain, dark urine, and jaundice. These symptoms usually last less than 2 months, but some people continue to experience symptoms for up to 6 months. Although death due to hepatitis A infection is not common, patients may require hospitalization. There is no cure for hepatitis A, but patients should be given supportive care, including bed rest, fluids, and antipyretics (CDC, 2008b).

Prevention using the hepatitis A vaccine is the key for hepatitis A infections. Hepatitis A vaccine is recommended for:

- All children 1 year (12 through 23 months) of age
- Persons 1 year of age and older traveling to or working in countries with a high or intermediate prevalence of Hepatitis A
- Children and adolescents through 18 years of age who live in states or communities where routine vaccination has been implemented because of high disease incidence
- Men who have sexual contact with other men
- Persons who use street drugs
- Persons with chronic liver disease
- Persons who are treated with clotting factor concentrates
- Persons who work with HAV-infected primates or who work with HAV in research laboratories (CDC 2008b)

Hepatitis B Vaccine

Hepatitis B is a liver disease caused by the hepatitis B virus (HBV). The spread of HBV occurs through contact with blood that contains the hepatitis B virus. This can occur through having sex with an HBV-infected person without using a condom or by sharing needles for intravenous drug use. Other ways to transmit HBV include tattooing and body piercing with contaminated needles, sharing razors or toothbrushes with an infected person, during birth from an infected mother to her child, and needlestick or sharps injuries in health care workers. Most people with acute hepatitis B have signs or symptoms when infected with HBV, but some patients may be asymptomatic. For example, children younger than 5 years who become infected rarely show any symptoms. Signs and symptoms of hepatitis B infection can include nausea, anorexia, fatigue, myalgias, arthralgias, and abdominal pain. Some patients may also report dark urine, light-colored stools, and jaundice. Hepatitis B can be very serious. Some people who are infected with HBV may be unable to clear the virus and become chronically infected. Although the signs and symptoms of HBV infection resolve, these patients remain infectious and can transmit HBV to others. Patients with chronic infection are at high risk of developing chronic liver disease, including cirrhosis, liver failure, and liver cancer (CDC, 2008c).

Prevention of hepatitis B infection can be achieved by vaccination. The hepatitis B vaccine series is a sequence of shots that stimulates a person's natural immune system to protect against HBV. After the vaccine is given, the body makes antibodies that protect a person against the virus. An antibody is a substance found in the blood that is produced in response to a virus invading the body. These antibodies are then stored in the body and will fight off the infection if a person is exposed to the hepatitis B virus in the future (CDC, 2008c).

Hepatitis B vaccination is recommended for:

- All infants, starting with the first dose of hepatitis B vaccine at birth
- All children and adolescents younger than 19 years of age who have not been vaccinated
- People whose sex partners have hepatitis B
- Sexually active persons who are not in a long-term, mutually monogamous relationship
- Persons seeking evaluation or treatment for a sexually transmitted disease
- Men who have sexual contact with other men
- People who share needles, syringes, or other drug-injection equipment
- People who have close household contact with someone infected with the hepatitis B virus
- Health care and public safety workers at risk for exposure to blood or blood-contaminated materials or body fluids on the job
- People with end-stage renal disease, including predialysis, hemodialysis, peritoneal dialysis, and home dialysis patients
- Residents and staff of facilities for developmentally disabled persons
- Travelers to regions with moderate or high rates of Hepatitis B
- People with chronic liver disease

- People with HIV infection
- Anyone who wishes to be protected from hepatitis B virus infection (CDC, 2008c)

In order to reach individuals at risk for hepatitis B, vaccination is also recommended for anyone in or seeking treatment from the following:

- Sexually transmitted disease treatment facilities
- HIV testing and treatment facilities
- Facilities providing drug-abuse treatment and prevention services
- Health care settings targeting services to injection drug users
- Health care settings targeting services to men who have sex with men
- Chronic hemodialysis facilities and end-stage renal disease programs
- Correctional facilities
- Institutions and nonresidential day care facilities for developmentally disabled persons (CDC, 2008c)

All children should get their first dose of hepatitis B vaccine at birth. Two subsequent doses are usually administered over a 6-month period and completed by 6 to 18 months of age.

All children and adolescents younger than 19 years of age who have not yet gotten the vaccine should also be vaccinated. "Catch-up" vaccination is recommended for children and adolescents who were never vaccinated or who did not get the entire vaccine series. Any adult who is at risk for hepatitis B virus infection or who wants to be vaccinated should talk to a health professional about getting the vaccine series.

Herpes Zoster Vaccine

The *varicella zoster* virus (VZV) is responsible for both chickenpox and shingles (see Figure 3.1). After a person has had chickenpox, the virus rests in the body's nerves permanently. Approximately one-third of people who have been infected with chickenpox will later develop herpes zoster, commonly known as shingles. Shingles occurs when latent VZV reactivates and causes recurrent disease. The risk of getting shingles is highest in the elderly and in immunocompromised patients. Shingles usually starts as a painful rash with blisters that scab after 3 to 5 days. The rash and pain usually occur in a band on one side of the body, or clustered on one side of the face. The rash typically clears within 2 to 4 weeks. Before the rash develops, there is often pain, itching, or tingling in the area where the rash will develop. Other symptoms of shingles can include fever, headache, chills, and upset stomach. The most common complication of shingles is post-herpetic neuralgia (PHN). In patients with PHN, severe pain can continue after the rash has disappeared. The pain can be described as sharp or throbbing, and the skin may be unusually sensitive to touch and to changes in temperature. PHN can last for months or even years. Other rare complications include pneumonia, hearing problems, blindness, scarring, encephalitis, or death (CDC, 2008a).

FIGURE 3.1

Herpes zoster infection

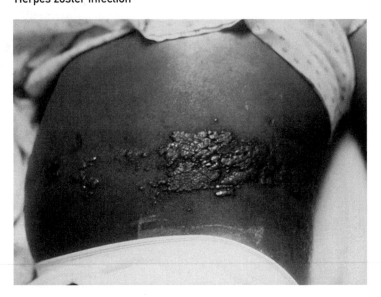

Courtesy of the Centers for Disease Control and Prevention.

In 2006, a vaccine for the prevention of herpes zoster was marketed. It is recommended that a single dose of the herpes zoster vaccine be administered to all adults age 60, including persons who have already had an episode of shingles.

H1N1 Vaccine

Information regarding the H1N1 influenza and the influenza virus vaccine can be found in Chapter 14.

Human Papillomavirus Vaccine (HPV) Vaccine

Human papillomavirus (HPV) is a group of more than 100 different viruses. These viruses usually infect the genital area and are spread through sexual contact. Some of these viruses can cause abnormal Pap tests and can lead to cancers of the cervix, vulva, vagina, anus, or penis. Other HPVs cause genital warts. HPV is the most common sexually transmitted infection in the United States. Approximately 20 million people are currently infected with HPV. At least 50% of sexually active men and women acquire genital HPV infection at some point in their lives. Most infected persons have no symptoms and unintentionally transmit the virus to a sex partner. Some infected people get visible genital warts or have precancerous changes in the cervix, vulva, anus, or penis. Most HPV infections eventually go away because the body's immune system eradicates the virus. However, about 10% of women infected with HPV develop persistent HPV infection and are at risk for developing precancerous lesions and cervical cancer, which can be fatal (CDC, 2010a).

In order to reduce the incidence of cervical cancer, the HPV vaccine was developed. HPV vaccine is routinely recommended for girls 11 to 12 years of age. It is important for girls to get HPV vaccine before their first sexual contact. HPV vaccine is given as a three-dose series: following the initial dose, a second dose 2 months after dose one, and a third dose is administered 6 months after dose one. HPV vaccine may be given at the same time as other vaccines. It is anticipated that this vaccine will soon be approved for use in boys, as well (CDC, 2010a).

Influenza Vaccine

A complete discussion of influenza and the influenza virus vaccine can be found in Chapter 14.

Meningococcal Vaccines

Meningococcal disease is caused by the bacterium *Neisseria meningitidis*. This bacterium has at least 13 different subtypes, but five, A, B, C, Y, and W-135, are responsible for almost all invasive disease. *N. meningitidis* is spread person-to-person through the exchange of respiratory and throat secretions such as by coughing, kissing, or sharing eating utensils. Meningococcal bacteria can produce life-threatening septicemia meningitis. Meningococcal disease progresses rapidly, so accurate diagnosis and immediate treatment is key. The most common symptoms of meningococcal infection are high fever, chills, lethargy, and a rash. In cases of meningitis, symptoms can also include headache, neck stiffness, and seizures. In an overwhelming number of meningococcal infections, shock, coma, and death can occur, even with appropriate medical treatment. Meningococcal disease is life-threatening, and approximately 9% to 12% of patients with meningococcal disease die despite appropriate antibiotic treatment. Of those who recover, up to 20% suffer from some serious after-effect, such as permanent hearing loss, limb loss, or brain damage (CDC, 2008e).

A vaccine containing the antigens for the most deadly subtypes of *N. meningitides* (A, C, Y, or W-135) is available. One dose of MCV4 is recommended for children and adolescents 11 through 18 years of age. This dose is normally given during the routine preadolescent immunization visit (at 11–12 years). Meningococcal vaccine should also be considered for people at increased risk for meningococcal disease, including

- College freshmen living in dormitories
- Microbiologists who are routinely exposed to meningococcal bacteria
- U.S. military recruits
- Anyone traveling to, or living in, a part of the world where meningococcal disease is common, such as parts of Africa
- Anyone who has a damaged spleen, or whose spleen has been removed

- Anyone who has a deficiency of the terminal component of the complement system
- People who might have been exposed to meningitis during an outbreak (CDC, 2008e)

Another meningococcal vaccine, the MPSV4 vaccine is made from the outer polysaccharide capsule of the meningococcal bacteria. This vaccine is used in adults over the age of 55 years. In clinical trials, it has been found that the MCV4 is as effective as MPSV4, but the MCV4 provides a longer duration of immunity. Consequently, although the MCV4 is the preferred vaccine for people 2 through 55 years of age in these risk groups, MPSV4 can be substituted if MCV4 is not available (CDC, 2008e).

Measles (Rubeola) Vaccine

Measles is caused by a virus that is spread through the air by infectious droplets and is highly contagious. Symptoms include fever, rhinitis, cough, anorexia, conjunctivitis, and a rash (Figure 3.2). The rash usually lasts 5 to 6 days and begins at the hairline, moves to the face and upper neck, and proceeds down the body. Measles can be a serious disease, with 30% of reported cases experiencing one or more complications. Death from measles occurred in approximately 2 per 1,000 reported cases in the United States from 1985 through 1992. Complications from measles are more common among very young children (younger than 5 years of age) and adults (older than 20 years of age). Diarrhea is the most common complication of measles (occurring in 8% of cases), especially in young children. Ear infections occur in 7% of reported cases. Pneumonia, occurring in 6%

FIGURE 3.2

Picture of child with measles

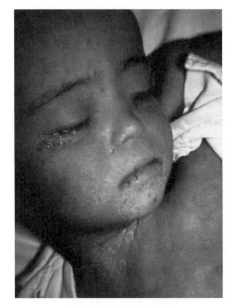

Courtesy of the Centers for Disease Control and Prevention / Dr. John Noble, Jr.

of reported cases, accounts for 60% of measles-related deaths. Approximately 1 out of 1,000 cases will develop acute encephalitis. This serious complication can lead to permanent brain damage. Measles during pregnancy increases the risk of premature labor, miscarriage, and low-birth-weight infants, although birth defects have not been linked to measles exposure. Measles can be especially severe in persons with compromised immune systems. There is no specific treatment for measles. People with measles need bed rest, fluids, and control of fever. Patients with complications may need treatment specific to their problem.

Although an individual measles vaccine is available, it is recommended that immunization for measles be accomplished through administration of the MMR vaccine (see following section).

Measles, Mumps, Rubella (MMR) Vaccine

For a description of the individual diseases, see the corresponding sections.

Immunization for measles, mumps, and rubella is available in a single, combination vaccine. The recommended schedule for this vaccine is two doses of MMR vaccine. The first dose is administered at 12 to 15 months of age, and a subsequent booster dose is given at 4 to 6 years of age. In certain cases, vaccination of adults with MMR may be warranted. For example, persons 18 years of age or older who were born after 1956 should get at least one dose of MMR vaccine, unless they have proof that they have been vaccinated or have had the diseases (CDC, 2008d).

Mumps

Mumps is caused by a virus. Mumps spreads from person to person through the air. It is less contagious than measles or chickenpox. The most common initial symptoms are nonspecific symptoms such as headache, anorexia, and a low-grade fever. Patients may also develop parotitis (Figure 3.3).

FIGURE 3.3

Picture of child with parotitis

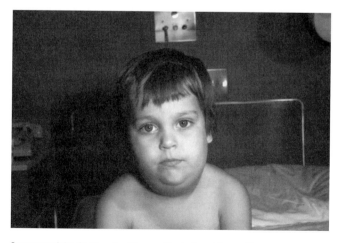

Courtesy of the Centers for Disease Control and Prevention.

In children, mumps is usually a mild disease. But in adults, the disease can be more serious. Complications can include meningitis and orchitis. Up to one-half of adolescent and adult men develop orchitis. This may involve pain, swelling, nausea, vomiting, and fever, with tenderness of the area possibly lasting for weeks. Approximately half of patients with orchitis have some degree of testicular atrophy, but sterility is uncommon. An increase in spontaneous abortion or miscarriage is seen in women who develop mumps during the first trimester of pregnancy. Deafness, in one or both ears, has also been reported.

Although an individual mumps vaccine is available, it is recommended that immunization for measles be accomplished through administration of the MMR vaccine (see "MMR vaccine").

Pneumococcal Conjugate Vaccine/ Pneumococcal Polysaccharide Vaccine

Pneumococcal disease is caused by the bacterium *Streptococcus pneumonia*. Although there are more than 90 subtypes, only a few produce the majority of invasive pneumococcal infections. The disease is spread from person to person by droplets in the air. Pneumococcal disease is a serious disease that causes much sickness and death. In fact, pneumococcal disease kills more people in the United States each year than all other vaccine-preventable diseases combined. There are three major conditions caused by invasive pneumococcal disease: pneumonia, bacteremia, and meningitis. Pneumococcal pneumonia is the most common disease caused by pneumococcal bacteria. Symptoms of pneumococcal pneumonia include the sudden onset of fever, rigors, chest pain, cough, dyspnea, tachycardia, tachypnea, and weakness. Pneumococcal bacteremia is the most common clinical presentation among children younger than 2 years. Finally, pneumococcal meningitis is responsible for up to 20% of all cases of bacterial meningitis in the United States. Symptoms of pneumococcal meningitis can include headache, tiredness, vomiting, irritability, fever, seizures, and coma. Pneumococcal meningitis can be fatal. Pneumococci are also a common cause of acute otitis media (CDC, 2010b).

There are two types of pneumococcal vaccine: pneumococcal polysaccharide vaccine and pneumococcal conjugate vaccine. The first pneumococcal polysaccharide vaccine was licensed in the United States in 1977. In 1983, an improved pneumococcal polysaccharide vaccine was licensed that contains purified protein from 23 types of pneumococcal bacteria (the old formulation contained 14 types). This pneumococcal polysaccharide vaccine is commonly known as PPSV23. The PPSV23 vaccine is licensed for use in adults and persons with certain risk factors who are 2 years and older. It should be administered to:

- All adults age 65 years or older
- Anyone age 2 years or older who has a long-term health problem such as cardiovascular disease, sickle cell anemia, alcoholism, lung disease, diabetes, cirrhosis, or leaks of cerebrospinal fluid
- Anyone who has or is getting a cochlear implant
- Anyone age 2 years or older who has a disease or condition that lowers the body's resistance to infection, such as Hodgkin's disease, kidney failure,

nephrotic syndrome, lymphoma, leukemia, multiple myeloma, HIV infection or AIDS, damaged spleen or no spleen, or organ transplant

■ Anyone age 2 years or older who is taking any drug or treatment that lowers the body's resistance to infection, such as long-term steroids, certain cancer drugs, or radiation therapy

■ Adults ages 19–64 who have asthma

■ Adults ages 19–64 who smoke cigarettes

■ In special situations, public health authorities may recommend the use of PPSV23 after PCV7 for Alaska Native or American Indian children ages 24 through 59 months who are living in areas in which risk of invasive pneumococcal disease is increased.

■ In special situations, public health authorities may recommend PPSV23 for Alaska Natives and American Indians ages 50 through 64 years who are living in areas in which the risk of invasive pneumococcal disease is increased (CDC, 2010b).

The pneumococcal conjugate vaccine was licensed in early 2000 and is used in preventing pneumococcal disease in infants and young children (from age 6 weeks to the 5th birthday). It is commonly known as PCV7 and should be administered to all infants. All infants and toddlers should get four doses of PCV7 vaccine, usually given at 12–15 months, 2 years, 4 years, and 6 years (CDC, 2010b).

Poliomyelitis Vaccine

Polio is caused by a virus. It is usually spread by the fecal–oral route, although some cases may be spread directly via an oral-to-oral route. Surprisingly, 95% of all individuals infected with polio have no apparent symptoms. Another 4%–8% of infected individuals have symptoms of a minor, nonspecific nature, such as sore throat and fever, nausea, vomiting, and other common symptoms of any viral illness. About 1%–2% of infected individuals develop nonparalytic aseptic (viral) meningitis, with temporary stiffness of the neck, back, and/or legs. Less than 1% of all polio infections result in the classic "flaccid paralysis," where the patient is left with permanent weakness or paralysis of legs, arms, or both. Of persons with paralytic polio, about 2%–5% of children die, and up to 15%–30% of adults die (CDC, 2000).

The first polio vaccine was an inactivated, or killed, vaccine (IPV) developed by Dr. Jonas Salk and licensed in 1955. In 1961, a live attenuated vaccine (trivalent oral polio virus, OPV) was developed by Dr. Albert Sabin. In 1988, an enhanced-potency IPV formulation became available, and by 1997 it had become part of the routine schedule for infants and children, given in a sequential combination with OPV. In 2000, an all-IPV vaccine schedule was adopted in the United States. IPV is also available in combination with other vaccines (e.g., DTaP-HepB-IPV, DTaP-IPV/Hib, or DTaP-IPV) (CDC, 2000).

All infants should get this vaccine unless they have a medical condition. Because these vaccines have traces of antibiotics (OPV contains traces of streptomycin, bacitracin, and neomycin; IPV has traces of streptomycin and neomycin), patients who have an allergy to these antibiotics or any of the components of the vaccine should not be vaccinated. A primary series of IPV consists of three properly spaced doses, usually given at 2 months, 4 months, and 6 to 18 months. A booster dose is given at 4 to 6 years unless the primary series was given so late that the third dose was given on or after the fourth birthday. Most adults do not need polio vaccine because they were vaccinated as children. Three groups of adults are at higher risk and should consider polio vaccination:

1. People traveling to areas of the world where polio is common
2. Laboratory workers who might handle polio virus
3. Health care workers treating patients who could have polio (CDC, 2000)

Adults in these three groups who have never been vaccinated against polio should get three doses of IPV with the first dose given at any time, the second dose 1 to 2 months later, and the third dose 6 to 12 months after the second dose. Adults in these three groups who have had one or two doses of polio vaccine in the past should get the remaining one or two doses.

Rotavirus Vaccine

Rotavirus disease is caused by a virus, the rotavirus. Rotavirus is spread through the oral route. The virus is ingested and then infects the lining of the intestines. Rotavirus is very contagious, spreading easily from children who are already infected to other children and sometimes adults. Rotavirus are shed in the stool of infected persons, and the virus can be easily spread via contaminated hands and objects, such as toys. Rotavirus infection usually starts with fever, nausea, and vomiting, followed by diarrhea. These symptoms can last from 3 to 7 days. Rotavirus infection often leads to dehydration, electrolyte disturbances, and metabolic acidosis. This can sometimes be severe enough to require hospital-ization in infants and children. Rarely, the dehydration leads to death.

A vaccine to prevent rotavirus gastroenteritis was first licensed in August 1998, but it was withdrawn in 1999 because of its possible association with in-tussusception. In 2006 and 2008, the U.S. Food and Drug Administration (FDA) approved two new rotavirus vaccines. These vaccines are both live attenuated vaccines and are liquids that are given orally. These vaccines are recommended for all infants. Depending on the brand of vaccine used, two or three doses should be administered between the ages of 2 and 6 months. The first dose of either vac-cine can be given as early as age 6 weeks or as late as age 14 weeks, 6 days. Vac-cination should not be started for infants once they reach their 15-week birthday. There must be at least 4 weeks between doses, and all doses must be given by age 8 months (CDC, 2009b).

Rubella/Rubeola

Rubella (German measles) is caused by a virus. It is spread from person to person through the air. Rubella is contagious but less so than measles and chickenpox. Children with rubella usually develop a rash as the initial manifestation, which starts on the face and progresses down the body. Older children and adults usually suffer from low-grade fever, swollen glands in the neck or behind the ears, and upper respiratory infection before they develop a rash (see Figure 3.3). Adult women often develop pain and stiffness in their finger, wrist, and knee joints, which may last up to a month. Up to half of people infected with rubella virus have no symptoms at all. Rubella is usually a mild disease in children, but adults tend to have more complications. Adults can develop encephalitis, thrombocytopenia, and hemorrhage. The main concern with rubella disease, however, is the effect it has on an infected pregnant woman. Rubella infection in the first trimester of pregnancy can lead to fetal death, premature delivery, and serious birth defects known as congenital rubella syndrome (CRS). In this syndrome, the rubella virus attacks a fetus, resulting in some type of birth defect, such as deafness, eye defects, heart defects, or mental retardation.

Although an individual rubella vaccine is available, it is recommended that immunization for measles be accomplished through administration of the MMR vaccine (see "Measles" and "MMR Vaccine") (CDC, 1998b).

Varicella (Chickenpox) Vaccine

Chickenpox is caused by the varicella-zoster virus. It spreads from person to person by direct contact with the fluid from infected blisters or through the air by coughing or sneezing. It is highly contagious. It can also be spread through direct contact with a sore from a person with shingles. The most common symptoms of chickenpox are rash, fever, coughing, fussiness, headache, and anorexia. The rash usually develops on the scalp and body, and then spreads to the face, arms, and legs (see Figure 3.4). The rash usually forms 200 to 500 itchy blisters in several successive crops. The illness lasts about 5 to 10 days. While most cases of chickenpox are mild, deaths from chickenpox can occur. The most common complication is bacterial infection of the skin or other parts of the body,

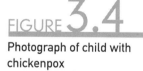

FIGURE 3.4

Photograph of child with chickenpox

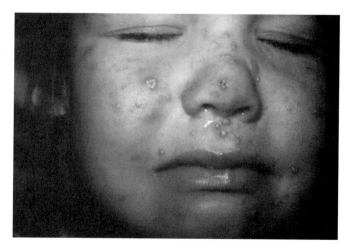

Courtesy of the Centers for Disease Control and Prevention / Dr. John Noble, Jr.

including the bones, lungs, joints, and blood. Rarely, the virus can also lead to pneumonia or infection of the brain (CDC, 2008a).

Children who have never had chickenpox should get two doses of chickenpox vaccine at 12–15 months of age and a booster dose at 4–6 years of age (which may be given earlier if at least 3 months after the first dose). In adolescents 13 years of age and older and adults (who have never had chickenpox or received the chickenpox vaccine, the vaccine is given as two doses administered at least 28 days apart (CDC, 2008a).

VACCINE SAFETY

After the FDA evaluates and deems a vaccine to be safe and effective, the vaccine is continually monitored for safety and efficacy. A list of currently available vaccines and their suggested routes of administration is provided in Table 3.1. As a result, the United States currently has the safest, most effective vaccines. However, there are risks associated with vaccination. Prior to the administration of any vaccine, the benefits and risks should be reviewed with the patient.

TABLE **3.1**

Vaccines Available in the U.S. and their Routes of Administration

IMMUNIZATION	METHOD OF ADMINISTRATION
Diphtheria-tetanus-acellular pertussis (DtAP)	Intramuscular
Diphtheria tetanus pertussis (DTP)	Intramuscular
DTaP-Hib conjugate	Intramuscular
Haemophilus influenza type b conjugate (Hib)	Intramuscular
Hepatitis A	Intramuscular
Hepatitis B	Intramuscular
Hepatitis C	Intramuscular
Hib conjugate-Hepatitis B	Intramuscular
Influenza	Intramuscular or intranasal
Meningococcal	Intramuscular or subcutaneous
Mumps	Subcutaneous
Pertussis	Intramuscular
Pneumococcal (polysaccharide; PPV)	Intramuscular or subcutaneous

(Continued)

TABLE **3.1**

(*Continued*)

IMMUNIZATION	METHOD OF ADMINISTRATION
Pneumococcal (polysaccharide-protein conjugate; PCV)	Intramuscular
Poliovirus vaccine, inactivated (IPV)	Subcutaneous
Rabies	Intramuscular or intradermal
Rotavirus	Oral
Rubella	Subcutaneous
Rubeola	Subcutaneous
Tetanus	Intramuscular
Tetanus–diphtheria (Td or DT)	Intramuscular
Tetanus and diphtheria toxoids and acellular pertussis (Tdap)	Intramuscular
Typhoid parenteral	Intramuscular
Typhoid (Ty21a)	Oral
Varicella	Subcutaneous
Yellow fever	Subcutaneous

From the Centers for Disease Control and Prevention.

Patients should be given the most updated version of the vaccine information statement (VIS). VISs are information sheets produced by the CDC that explain to vaccine recipients, their parents, or their legal representatives both the benefits and risks of a vaccine. Federal law requires that VISs be handed out before each dose of certain vaccinations are given. VISs are available at http://www.cdc.gov/vaccines/pubs/vis/default.htm#multi. In addition, the parent or patient should be asked if they have any allergies to ensure there are no contraindications to the vaccine (see http://www.immunize.org/catg.d/p3072a.pdf for a list of contraindications). All adverse reactions with vaccines should be reported to the FDA using the Vaccine Adverse Event Reporting System or VAERS (http://vaers.hhs.gov).

POST-TEST QUESTIONS

3-1. Which of the following vaccines is considered a live vaccine?
    a. Hemophilus influenza
    b. Hepatitis B

     c. Pneumococcal

     d. Varicella

3-2. Live vaccines may be contraindicated in patients with:

     a. Immunosuppression

     b. Growth hormone deficiency

     c. Allergy to thimerosal

     d. A previous reaction to pertussis vaccine

3-3. Which of the following is not a route of administration for common vaccines?

     a. Subcutaneous

     b. Intramuscular

     c. Oral

     d. Intravenous

3-4. Which of the following populations is at high risk of being exposed to the hepatitis B virus and therefore should be immunized?

     a. College freshmen living in dormitories

     b. U.S. military recruits

     c. Health care workers

     d. Adults ages 19–64 who have asthma

3-5. Which of the following vaccines is designed to prevent shingles?

     a. Pneumococcal vaccine

     b. Hepatitis A vaccine

     c. Human papillomavirus vaccine

     d. Herpes zoster vaccine

References

Centers for Disease Control and Prevention. (1998a). *Haemophilus Influenzae Type b (Hib) Vaccine.* Retrieved July 16, 2009, from http://www.cdc.gov/vaccines/vpd-vac/hib/default.htm

Centers for Disease Control and Prevention. (1998b). Measles, mumps, and rubella—Vaccine use and strategies for elimination of measles, rubella, and congenital rubella syndrome and control of mumps. Morbidity and Mortality Weekly Report, 47(RR-8). Retrieved November 8, 2010, from http://www.cdc.gov/mmwr/preview/mmwrhtml/00053391.htm

Centers for Disease Control and Prevention. (2000). *Polio vaccine.* Retrieved July 16, 2009, from http://www.cdc.gov/vaccines/vpd-vac/polio/default.htm

Centers for Disease Control and Prevention. (2006a). General recommendations on immunization. *Morbidity and Mortality Weekly Report, 55*(RR-15). Retrieved July 15, 2009, from http://www.cdc.gov/mmwr/PDF/rr/rr5515.pdf

Centers for Disease Control and Prevention. (2006b). Preventing tetanus, diphtheria, and pertussis among adults: Use of tetanus toxoid, reduced diphtheria toxoid and acellular pertussis vaccine. Morbidity and Mortality Weekly Report, 55(RR-17). Retrieved November 8, 2010, from http://www.cdc.gov/mmwr/PDF/rr/rr5517.pdf

Centers for Disease Control and Prevention. (2007). *Vaccines and preventable diseases: Pertussis (whooping cough) vaccination.* Retrieved July 16, 2009, from http://www.cdc.gov/vaccines/vpd-vac/pertussis/default.htm#vacc

Centers for Disease Control and Prevention. (2008a). *Chickenpox vaccine.* Retrieved July 17, 2009, from http://www.cdc.gov/vaccines/vpd-vac/varicella/default.htm

Centers for Disease Control and Prevention. (2008b). *Hepatitis A vaccination.* Retrieved July 16, 2009, from http://www.cdc.gov/vaccines/vpd-vac/hepa/default.htm

Centers for Disease Control and Prevention. (2008c). *Hepatitis B vaccination.* Retrieved July 16, 2009, from http://www.cdc.gov/vaccines/vpd-vac/hepb/default.htm

Centers for Disease Control and Prevention. (2008d). *Measles, mumps, and rubella (MMR) vaccines.* Retrieved July 16, 2009, from http://www.cdc.gov/vaccines/pubs/vis/downloads/vis-mmr.pdf

Centers for Disease Control and Prevention. (2008e). *Meningococcal vaccines.* Retrieved July 16, 2009, from http://www.cdc.gov/vaccines/vpd-vac/mening/default.htm

Centers for Disease Control and Prevention. (2008f). Prevention of herpes zoster. Morbidity and Mortality Weekly Report, 57(RR-5). Retrieved November 8, 2010, from http://www.cdc.gov/mmwr/PDF/rr/rr5705.pdf

Centers for Disease Control and Prevention. (2009a). *Vaccine safety and adverse events.* Retrieved July 15, 2010, from http://www.cdc.gov/vaccines/vac-gen/safety/default.htm

Centers for Disease Control and Prevention. (2009b). Prevention of rotavirus gastroenteritis among infants and children. Morbidity and Mortality Weekly Report, 58(RR-2). Retrieved November 8, 2010, from http://www.cdc.gov/mmwr/PDF/rr/rr5802.pdf

Centers for Disease Control and Prevention. (2010a). *HPV vaccine.* Retrieved July 15, 2010, from http://cdc.gov/vaccines/vpd-vac/hpv/default.htm

Centers for Disease Control and Prevention. (2010b). *Pneumococcal conjugate vaccine.* Retrieved July 15, 2010, from http://cdc.gov/vaccines/vpd-vac/pneumo/default.htm

World Health Organization. (2010). *Immunization.* Retrieved July 15, 2009, from http://www.who.int/topics/immunization/en

Web Sites

http://www.aap.org
http://www.aafp.org
http://www.cdc.gov/nip/acip
http://www.cdc.gov/vaccines/ed/encounter08/downloads/Table6.pdf
http://phil.cdc.gov/phil/home.asp
http://vaers.hhs.gov

Infection Control in the Community Health Care Setting

4

This chapter includes topics on proper nursing bag technique, including the cleansing of equipment in the home setting. The content differentiates between critical and noncritical equipment. The steps for cleaning urinary catheters using the boiling and microwave methods are reviewed. There is discussion on home-generated medical waste and sharp disposal in the home. Patient and family education in the home setting is reviewed. This includes care of the foley catheter, leg bag care, and care of closed urinary drainage systems. Catheter-associated urinary tract infections are discussed. Finally, post mortem care in the home is discussed.

OBJECTIVES

1. List topics that should be discussed when educating a family about standard precautions.
2. List four principles regarding proper bag technique.
3. Differentiate between critical and noncritical equipment, and explain how this affects the storage and cleaning.
4. List the steps for cleaning a urinary catheter using the boiling and microwave methods.
5. Differentiate between regulated medical waste and home-generated medical waste.

PRE-TEST QUESTIONS

4-1. Which of the following is true about proper bag technique?
    a. Place the bag on a clean, dry surface away from small children and pets.
    b. Place the bag on the floor so it is not in anyone's way.
    c. If the inside or outside of the bag becomes significantly soiled, wash the bag with bleach and hang to dry.
    d. The inside of the bag should be cleaned on a regular basis by removing the inside items and cleaning with soap and water.

4-2. Which of the following is true?
    a. Critical items must be kept covered, but not sealed, while inside the bag.
    b. Semicritical items are items that contact intact skin.
    c. Items that may come in contact with intact skin must be sterile.
    d. Noncritical items should be cleaned with low level disinfectant, such as 60% to 90% isopropyl alcohol.

4-3. When using the boiling method for intermittent urinary catheter cleaning, which of the following are true?
    a. Cleanse the catheter with povidone-iodine on the inside and outside, rinse with tap water.
    b. Boil for 5 minutes.
    c. Dry on a clean paper towel and allow to cool before use.
    d. Store in isopropyl alcohol in a clean, closeable container.

4-4. Caregivers should be instructed to wear gloves in all of the following situations EXCEPT:
    a. Whenever dealing with blood or body fluids
    b. Whenever coming in contact with intact skin
    c. Whenever applying topical medications or skin emollients
    d. Whenever coming in contact with contaminated items

4-5. Home-generated medical waste includes:
    a. Empty prescription vials
    b. Used tissues
    c. Used syringes
    d. Clothes soiled with fecal material

Infection control and prevention in the home care or hospice setting presents unique challenges to health care workers (HCW). Unlike acute care, long-term care, or outpatient facilities, HCWs who care for clients in their homes have little to no control over the environment in which they provide care. Home care professionals must adjust to different environments throughout their day. Their role entails not only practicing infection control measures to protect themselves but also to be diligent in the education of their clients about the importance of infection control and prevention.

STANDARD PRECAUTIONS

HCWs who practice in the home care setting must follow standard precautions, which include the use of hand hygiene and personal protective equipment

(PPE) such as gloves, gown, mask, eye protection, and face shield, depending on the anticipated exposure (see chapter 2, "Bloodborne Pathogen Standard"). They must also keep an adequate supply of PPE with them at all times. If an item is used, it should be replenished as soon as possible. Home care professionals are not always aware of what types of environments they are entering and therefore need to be prepared for any situation that may arise.

Education is one of the most important, if not the most important, functions of the home care professional. Patients, their family members, and their other caregivers need to understand when and why standard precautions should be used. Caregivers may fail to realize that they need to protect themselves and others when caring for a loved one.

EDUCATION POINTS FOR CAREGIVERS

1. Hand hygiene should be performed
   * Regardless of health status
   * Before and after patient care contact
   * Whenever hands become visibly soiled
   * After removing gloves
2. Gloves should be worn
   * Whenever dealing with blood or body fluids
   * Whenever coming in contact with contaminated items or nonintact skin
   * Whenever applying topical medications or skin emollients
3. Respiratory hygiene should be practiced
   * To prevent the transmission of respiratory infections
   * Whenever caregivers have signs of illness, including cough, congestion, rhinorrhea, or increased respiratory secretions
   * By covering the mouth/nose with a tissue when coughing, with prompt disposal of used tissues and implementing hand hygiene thereafter
   * By coughing into their sleeve rather than their hands if a tissue is not available
   * By wearing a surgical mask if tolerated
   * By maintaining spatial separation from others, ideally over 3 feet, if signs and symptoms of respiratory infection are present. (Siegel, Rhinehart, Jackson, Chiarello, & the Healthcare Infection Control Practices Advisory Committee [HICPAC], 2007)

TRANSMISSION-BASED PRECAUTIONS

The information guiding the decision to place a home care or hospice patient on transmission-based precautions should be outlined in the home care or hospice organization's patient care policies and procedures. It should not be dependent on a physicians order. The need for transmission-based precautions (see Chapter 1, "Basic Infection Control") should be determined based on report of the patient's history or current condition from a referral source, or based on assessments made any time during the course of care (Rhinehart & McGoldrick, 2006).

Isolation in the community setting entails an assessment of the patient's surroundings and determination of who lives with the patient and who cares for the patient. When all of the individuals who have contact with the patient are identified, these people should receive education regarding appropriate precautions. If a patient requires transmission-based precautions, the patient should be contained in his or her own room and provided access to a separate bathroom. If this is not possible, additional cleaning and disinfection need to be taken to protect family members and/or caregivers.

Transmission-Based Precautions Education

1. Hand hygiene
2. When and how to use PPE
3. Modes of transmission
4. Duration of infectivity
5. Cleaning and disinfecting measures for the home environment
6. Strategies to prevent the transmission of infection when the patient must leave the home.
   a. For example, a patient should wear a surgical mask when going to a doctor's appointment if a cough is present.

The home care clinician should also be diligent in communicating information regarding transmission-based precautions while being mindful of patient confidentially. The information should be placed in the clinical record and care plan and communicated to other staff who will be involved in the care of the client (Rhinehart & McGoldrick, 2006). Communication keeps everyone involved protected.

PROPER BAG TECHNIQUE

Home care HCWs are required to bring a nursing bag into the home. This bag typically contains all medical equipment needed during the home care visit. Proper bag technique is an essential component of infection control.

The Principles of Proper Bag Technique

- Choose a bag constructed of washable fabric with multiple compartments for storage.
- Place the bag on a clean, dry, upholstered surface away from small children and pets. Never place the bag on the floor.
- If the inside or outside of the bag becomes significantly soiled, wash the bag with hot soapy water, rinse, and place in a dryer or hang dry.
- The inside of the bag should be cleaned on a regular basis by removing the inside items and cleaning with a disinfectant wipe.
- Perform hand hygiene before reaching into the bag. If the bag needs to be accessed after patient care is performed, gloves should be removed and hands washed to prevent contamination (see Figure 4.1).

FIGURE 4.1
Checking expiration date of liquid hand gel (alcohol rub) in the home setting

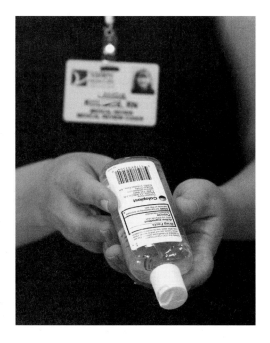

- Items or devices that enter sterile tissue or spaces (critical items) must be kept sterile while inside the bag and should be kept in their sterile wrappers (see Figure 4.2).
  - Examples of critical items include injection needles and urinary catheters.

- Items that contact mucus membranes or nonintact skin (semicritical items) should be kept covered while inside the bag.
  - Examples of semicritical items include respiratory equipment such as a nasal cannula.

- Items that may come in contact with intact skin (noncritical items) should be cleaned with low level disinfection, such as 60% to 90% isopropyl alcohol, before being placed back in the bag.
  - Examples of noncritical items include stethoscopes and blood pressure cuffs. (Rhinehart & McGoldrick, 2006)

Whenever possible, patient-care equipment, such as a blood pressure cuff, should be left in the home until discharge from home care services, or the patient should purchase their own (see Figures 4.3–4.7). If noncritical patient-care equipment cannot remain in the home, it should be cleaned and disinfected with a low- to intermediate-level disinfectant before it is placed into the nursing bag. Alternatively, place contaminated reusable items in a plastic bag for transport (Centers for Disease Control and Prevention [CDC], 2007).

FIGURE 4.2

Nursing bag set-up

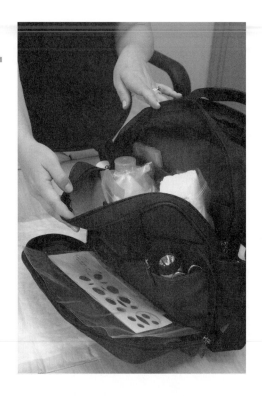

FIGURE 4.3

Dirty area of nursing bag
(includes stethoscope and
blood pressure cuff)

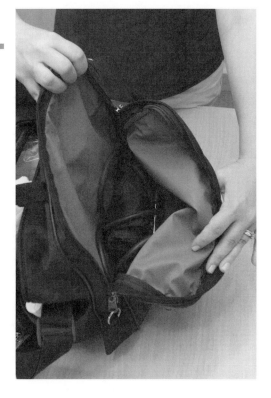

FIGURE 4.4

Remove stethoscope from bag prior to use

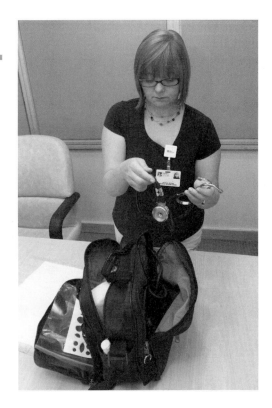

FIGURE 4.5

Cleanse stethoscope with alcohol wipe

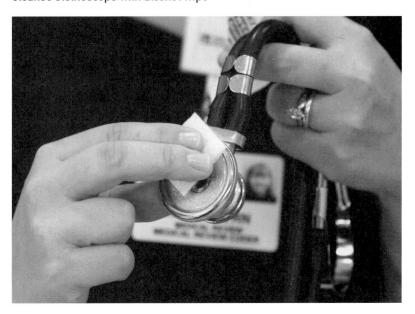

FIGURE 4.6

Perform vital signs after properly cleansing stethoscope

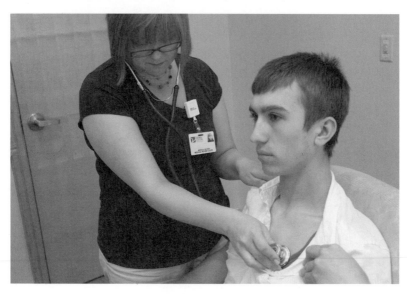

FIGURE 4.7

Cleanse stethoscope after use

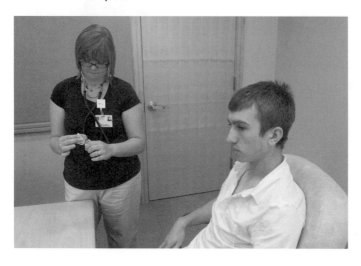

MEDICAL WASTE AND SHARP DISPOSAL

There is a distinction between regulated medical waste and home-generated medical waste. *Home-generated medical waste* is created through the administration of injectable medication and other invasive or noninvasive procedures. It includes, but is not limited to, syringes, needles with attached tubing, and other materials. Home-generators of medical waste include any individual who produces waste as a result of medical care in the home through self-administration practices or by a family member or other person not receiving money for their services. It does NOT include waste produced by the HCW (New Jersey Department of Health and Senior Services, 2008). Medical waste generated by the HCW must be disposed of in a manner similar to the one outlined previously and must comply with federal, state, and local regulations. A directory of state agencies that are responsible for this regulation can be accessed at http://www.safenee dledisposal/org/resswl.html (Rhinehart & McGoldrick, 2006). The home care clinician must educate caregivers regarding proper disposal of home-generated medical waste, including the use of personal sharps containers. There are several options available to patients for the proper disposal of their syringes.

CATHETER-ASSOCIATED URINARY TRACT INFECTIONS

Catheter-associated urinary tract infection (CAUTI) is the most common health care–associated infection (HAI), comprising more that 40% of all HAIs. Proper management of the indwelling catheter can contribute to the prevention of these infections. The risk of acquiring a urinary tract infection (UTI) depends on the method and duration of catheterization, the quality of the catheter care, and the host susceptibility. Host factors that increase the risk for a UTI include advanced age, female gender, general debilitation, colonization of the meatus by urinary pathogens, and bowel incontinence (Rhinehart & McGoldrick, 2006) (see Figures 4.8–4.10).

Microorganisms that inhabit the meatus or distal urethra can enter the urinary tract when the urinary catheter is inserted. After catheter insertion, infectious organisms may migrate along the outside of the catheter in the periurethral mucous sheath or along the internal lumen of the catheter if the urinary collection system becomes contaminated.

For patients requiring indwelling urethral catheterization, adherence to a sterile continuously closed system of urinary drainage is the cornerstone of infection control. All other interventions can be viewed as adjunctive measures because none have proven to be as effective in reducing the frequency of CAUTIs.

CDC Recommendations for Preventing Infections in Patients with Urinary Catheters

- Insertion and maintenance of the catheter should be handled by those individuals who know the correct technique.

FIGURE 4.8

Place a moisture barrier under patient prior to emptying leg bag

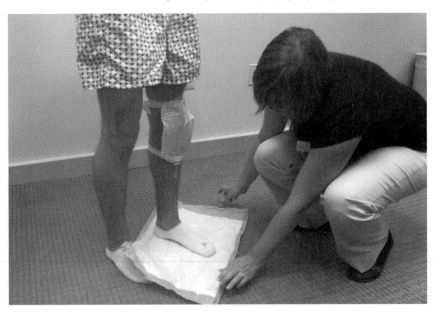

FIGURE 4.9

Emptying leg bag

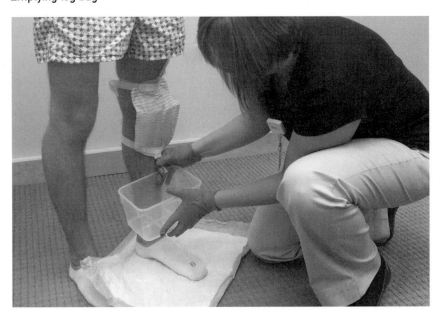

FIGURE **4.9**

Emptying the leg bag *(continued)*

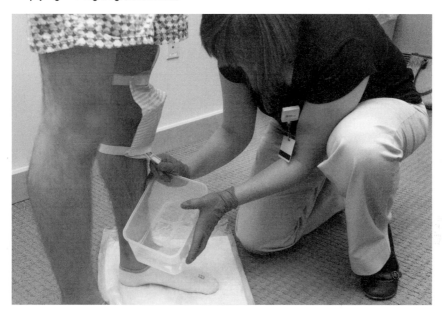

FIGURE **4.10**

Cleanse connection tube with alcohol prior to reconnecting

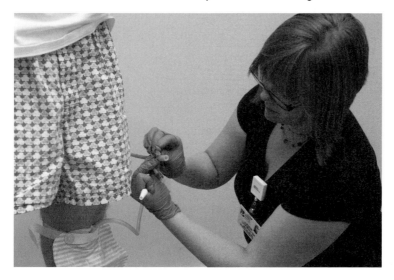

FIGURE 4.10

Cleanse connection tube with alcohol prior to reconnecting *(continued)*

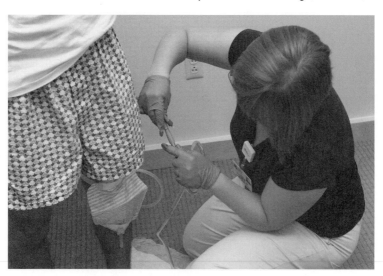

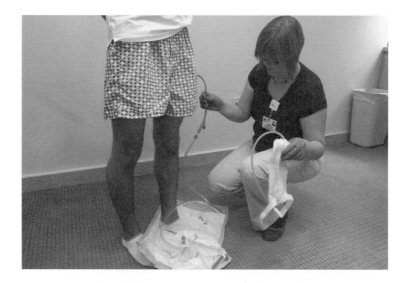

▧ Periodic in-services should be given to review the correct techniques and potential complications.

▧ Urinary catheters should be inserted only when necessary and left in place only for as long as necessary. They should not be used solely for the convenience of patient-care personnel.

- For selected patients, other methods of urinary drainage such as condom catheter drainage, suprapubic catheterization, and intermittent catheterization can be useful alternatives. Hand washing should be done immediately before and after any manipulation of the catheter site.
- Insertion should be done using aseptic technique and sterile equipment.
- Use the smallest catheter possible, consistent with good drainage, to minimize urethral trauma.
- Indwelling catheters should be properly secured after insertion to prevent movement and urethral traction.
- The catheter and drainage tube should not be disconnected unless the catheter must be irrigated.
- If breaks in aseptic technique occur, the system should be replaced using aseptic technique after disinfecting the catheter tubing junction.
- Irrigation should be avoided unless obstruction is anticipated as might occur with bleeding after prostatic or bladder surgery. An intermittent method of irrigation may be used for obstructions due to clots, mucus, or other causes. If frequent irrigations are needed the catheter should be changed if it is likely that the catheter itself is contributing to the problem.
- Achieve free flow of urine by keeping the catheter and collecting tube from kinking.
- The collection bag should be emptied regularly using a separate collecting container and should always be kept below the bladder. The draining spigot and nonsterile collecting container should never come in contact with each other.
- Regular bacteriologic monitoring of catheterized patients as an infection control measure has not been established and is not recommended.
- Prophylactic antibiotics are controversial and their routine use is not recommended. (CDC & HICPAC, 2009)

For patients with certain types of bladder emptying dysfunction, such as those caused by spinal cord injuries or other neurological disorders, intermittent catheterization is commonly used. The intermittent urethral catheter may be reused as long as the cleaning and disinfection process is performed effectively and does not change the structural integrity or function of the urethral catheter. Methods used by home care organization include either boiling or microwaving the catheter (Rhinehart & McGoldrick, 2006).

Methods for Cleaning and Disinfecting Intermittent Urinary Catheters

Boiling Method

- Cleanse the catheter with soap and tap water on the inside and outside, rinse with tap water.
- Boil for 15 minutes.
- Dry on a clean paper towel and allow to cool before use.
- Store in a clean, closeable container or a new plastic bag.

Microwaving Method

- Cleanse the catheter with soap and tap water on the inside and outside, rinse with tap water.
- Place in a bowl of water and microwave on high for 15 minutes.
- Dry on a clean paper towel and allow to cool before use.
- Store in a clean, closeable container or a new plastic bag.

POSTMORTEM CARE

In providing routine postmortem care and handling of the body postmortem, the home care HCW should maintain standard precautions and protect themselves from blood or body fluids as they would if the patient were still alive. However, if the patient was on transmission-based precautions prior to death, wearing a mask postmortem is not necessary.

If there is a concern that the patient's death was caused by an agent of bioterrorism, the following precautions should be taken in addition to standard ones:

- Droplet precautions for pneumonic plague
- Airborne precautions for smallpox
- Contact precautions for smallpox and viral hemorrhagic fever

The room in the home where the patient resided should be cleaned and disinfected, especially high touch items (e.g., doorknobs), and the linens used by the patient should be washed in hot soap and water. It is also important to communicate with the funeral home personnel or other individuals accepting possession of the body as to what precautions are needed (Rhinehart & McGoldrick, 2006).

POST-TEST QUESTIONS

4-1. Which of the following is true about proper bag technique?
   a. Place the bag on a clean, dry surface away from small children and pets.
   b. Place the bag on the floor so it is not in anyone's way.
   c. If the inside or outside of the bag becomes significantly soiled, wash the bag with bleach and hang to dry.
   d. The inside of the bag should be cleaned on a regular basis by removing the inside items and cleaning with soap and water.

4-2. Which of the following is true?
   a. Critical items must be kept covered, but not sealed, while inside the bag.
   b. Semicritical items are items that contact intact skin.
   c. Items that may come in contact with intact skin must be sterile.
   d. Noncritical items should be cleaned with low level disinfection, such as 60% to 90% isopropyl alcohol.

4-3. When using the boiling method for intermittent urinary catheter cleaning, which of the following is true?

    a. Cleanse the catheter with povidone-iodine on the inside and outside, rinse with tap water.

    b. Boil for 5 minutes.

    c. Dry on a clean paper towel and allow to cool before use.

    d. Store in isopropyl alcohol in a clean, closeable container.

4-4. Caregivers should be instructed to wear gloves in all of the following situations EXCEPT:

    a. Whenever dealing with blood or body fluids

    b. Whenever coming in contact with intact skin

    c. Whenever applying topical medications or skin emollients

    d. Whenever coming in contact with contaminated items

4-5. Home-generated medical waste includes:

    a. Empty prescription vials

    b. Used tissues

    c. Used syringes

    d. Clothes soiled with fecal material

References

Centers for Disease Control and Prevention. (2007). *Information about MRSA for healthcare personnel*. Retrieved July 15, 2010, from http://www.cdc.gov/ncidod/dhqp/ar_mrsa_health careFS.html

Centers for Disease Control and Prevention & the Healthcare Infection Control Practices Advisory Committee (HICPAC). (2009). Guideline for prevention of catheter-associated urinary tract infections. Retrieved July 15, 2010, from http://www.cdc.gov/hicpac/pdf/CAUTI/ CAUTIguideline2009final.pdf

New Jersey Department of Health and Senior Services. (2008). *Safe syringe disposal guide for home generated medical waste*. Retrieved July 15, 2010, from http://www.state.nj.us/health/ eoh/phss/syringe.pdf

Rhinehart, E., & McGoldrick, M. (2006). *Infection control in home care and hospice* (2nd ed.). Sudbury, MA: Jones and Bartlett Publishers.

Siegel, J.D., Rhinehart, E., Jackson, M., Chiarello, L., & the Healthcare Infection Control Practices Advisory Committee (HICPAC). (2007). *2007 Guideline for isolation precautions: Preventing transmission of infectious agents in healthcare settings*. Retrieved July 14, 2010, from http://www.cdc.gov/ncidod/dhqp/pdf/isolation2007.pdf

Web Sites

http://www.cdc.gov
http://www.lungusa.org
http://www.safeneedledisposal/org/resswl.html
http://www.state.nj.us

Outpatient Health Care Provider Offices

5

This chapter includes topics on infection control practices in the outpatient health care provider offices. The standards for disinfection, general housekeeping, sterilization, and waste disposal are reviewed. The content topics of point-of-care testing and the Spaulding Classification of Level of Processing are reviewed. There is discussion of evidence-based standards and education when there is a community outbreak. Finally, the World Health Organization guidelines for hand hygiene are discussed, as well as triaging of patients during an outbreak in the community.

OBJECTIVES

1. Describe infection control practices that should be followed in outpatient (OP) health care provider (HCP) offices.
2. Outline standards for disinfection, general housekeeping, sterilization, and waste disposal in OP HCP offices.
3. Discuss the Occupational Safety and Health Administration (OSHA) blood-borne pathogen standard as it pertains to OP HCP offices.
4. Define common OP HCP point-of-care testing (POCT) methods.
5. Discuss relevant resources available to HCPs and patients to provide evidence-based practice (EBP) standards and education for community outbreaks.

PRE-TEST QUESTIONS

5-1. Which of the following does NOT need to be disinfected or sterilized?
   a. Stethoscope
   b. Otoscope handle

    c. Computer keyboards
    d. Disposable thermometer

5-2. The process that destroys or eliminates all forms of microbial life and is carried out in health care facilities by physical or chemical methods is called:
    a. Cleaning
    b. High-level disinfection
    c. Low-level disinfection
    d. Sterilization

5-3. Which of the following is considered general waste or municipal waste?
    a. Sharps
    b. Soiled tissue
    c. Blood products
    d. Isolation waste

5-4. OSHA requires employers to offer which of the following vaccines to newly employed staff?
    a. Hepatitis A
    b. Hepatitis B
    c. Varicella zoster
    d. Meningococcal

5-5. An exposure control plan is a plan to:
    a. Minimize or eliminate exposure to bloodborne pathogens
    b. Describes the treatment necessary following a needlestick injury
    c. Should be updated every 3 to 5 years
    d. Should be distributed to all patients annually

    With the impetus to reduce health care costs, patients with acute illness are increasingly being managed in the OP setting. In light of this trend, the potential for spread of infection outside of the acute care hospital has increased. Infection control and prevention principles must be applied with the same rigor in both inpatient and outpatient settings to reduce the risk of exposure to patients and health care providers. This chapter discusses infection control and prevention principles and practice in the OP HCP office. As this environment of care is different from the hospital, information on current guidelines and recommendations for best infection control and prevention practices unique to this setting are reviewed.

CURRENT STANDARDS

Standards for infection control in the OP HCP office are outlined by the World Health Organization (WHO), OSHA, and the Centers for Disease Control and Prevention (CDC). Standards are continually revised and updated based on current evidence, so it is imperative that all OP HCP offices keep up-to-date on the most current standards. Web sites for these organizations are listed at the end of this chapter.

ASSESSMENT OF INFECTION CONTROL AND PREVENTION NEEDS IN THE OP OFFICE SETTING

The following questions may serve the practitioner well prior to new construction, leasing, or renovation of a new or existing office space as an initial assessment to ensure that office design and layout will facilitate best infection control practices:

- Am I serving a high risk population? If so, what are the needs of this population?
- What services/procedures will I be providing?
- What is the patient mix and patient case load?
- Do I need clean or soiled storage rooms?
- Am I storing sterile supplies near, under, or on surfaces that can get wet easily?
- Do I need more closed cupboards to store medical equipment?
- Can I have my reprocessing/sterilization room as a separate room clearly designed to separate the dirty side from the clean side, with enough counter space?
- Are there sufficient freestanding hand hygiene facilities available (sinks and/or waterless product dispensers)?
  - Are they in the waiting room, each examination room, washroom, laboratory area, medication preparation area, and soiled utility room?

- Is the waiting room big enough so that potentially infectious patients can be segregated?
- What is the potential work flow?
- Is the environment/furniture easy to clean?
- Is the garbage bin near the door? (The College of Physicians and Surgeons of Ontario, 2004)

The physical plant of the OP HCP office is the first challenge that must be addressed. Offices built in the 1980s were not typically designed to meet the standards of today's infection control environment. For example, flooring surfaces such as wood or linoleum are preferred to carpeting to facilitate ease of cleaning and disinfection (BC Centre for Disease Control [BCCDC], 2004). Furniture with cloth upholstery poses cleaning challenges so nonporous materials are preferred (American Academy of Pediatrics [AAP] Committee on Infectious Diseases, 2007).

Guidelines are published for the design and construction of health care facilities (HCFs) by the Facility Guidelines Institute (2006) of the American Institute of Architects (AIA) and include those appropriate to the OP medical office, diagnostic imaging centers, endoscopy suites, and other ambulatory care centers. These standards should be reviewed during the design process and incorporated into the final architectural design. Selected guidelines for OP facilities are summarized in Table 5.1.

TABLE 5.1

American Institute of Architects' Selected Guidelines for the Design and Construction of Health Care Facilities

Standards	
General considerations	Patient privacy, environment of care, ventilation, facility access, parking.
Diagnostic and treatment locations	Minimal net square foot requirements for general, special purpose, and treatment examination rooms; hand wash stations; clean storage; soiled holding; and supportive areas for examination and treatment rooms.
Service areas	Housekeeping rooms, sharps and medical waste collection, storage and disposal.
Administrative and public areas	Entrance, reception, public toilets and telephones, general or individual offices, equipment and supply storage, medical records.
Construction standards	Building codes, provisions for disasters, corridor width, ceiling height.

Adapted from *Guidelines for Design and Construction of Healthcare Facilities,* by The Facility Guidelines Institute, The American Institute of Architects Academy of Architecture for Health with the assistance from the U.S. Department of Health and Human Services, (2006). Washington, DC: American Institute of Architects.

After the structural design of the setting is deemed appropriate to ensure that proper infection control can be maintained within the physical location, infection control procedures must be developed to address the following:

- Standard precautions and hand hygiene
- Cleaning, disinfection, and sterilization, as appropriate
- Medical waste, specimen handling, and disposal
- Control of bloodborne pathogen exposure
- Surveillance and reporting activities for patients and staff (Pyrek, 2002)

STANDARD PRECAUTIONS AND HAND HYGIENE

Standard precautions (see Chapter 1, "Basic Infection Control") are based on the principle that all blood, body fluids, secretions, and excretions, except sweat, nonintact skin, and mucous membranes, may contain transmissible infectious agents. Standard precautions for infection control include a group of infection prevention practices that apply to all patients, regardless of suspected or confirmed infection status, in any setting in which health care is delivered (Siegel, Rhinehart, Jackson, Chiarello, & the Healthcare Infection Control Practices Advisory Committee [HICPAC], 2007).

TABLE 5.2

Hand Hygiene Recommendations

ORGANIZATION	HAND HYGIENE RECOMMENDATIONS	WEB SITE
AAP	Infection Prevention and Control in Pediatric Ambulatory Settings (2007)	http://pediatrics.aappublications.org/cgi/content/full/120/3/650
Association for Professionals in Infection Control (APIC) and CDC	Guidelines for Hand Hygiene in Health-Care Settings (2002)	http://www.cdc.gov/mmwr/PDF/rr/rr5116.pdf
OSHA	Healthcare wide hazards (page last updated 12/22/2008)	http://www.osha.gov/SLTC/etools/hospital/hazards/infection/infection.html
The Joint Commission (TJC)	Infection Control in Office Surgery (2009)	http://www.jcrinc.com/common/PDFs/fpdfs/pubs/pdfs/JCReqs/JCP-10-09-S4.pdf
WHO	WHO guidelines on Hand Hygiene in Healthcare (2009)	http://whqlibdoc.who.int/publications/2009/9789241597906_eng.pdf

As national and international organizations recognize hand hygiene as an effective method for prevention of infection, particular care should be exercised to ensure that space design includes this component as a priority (see Table 5.2).

To highlight global awareness to the need for improved hygiene practices, 2008 was designated as the International Year of Sanitization by the UN General Assembly. The first ever global hand-washing day took place on Wednesday, October 15, 2008.

Hand Hygiene, First and Last

Successful hand hygiene practice by health care workers (HCW) and office personnel is predicated upon ready access to appropriate supplies and sinks. Hand hygiene should be performed before any patient encounter. Sinks should be located in all clinical care areas, including examination rooms, restrooms, laboratory areas, and any other place where patient care is provided. Ideally, single faucet sinks should be utilized. Faucet aerators are not recommended because this type of faucet has been linked to contamination by *Pseudomonas* species and other bacteria (BCCDC, 2004). Soap dispensers should be alongside sinks and paper towels located within easy reach of the sink. Alcohol-based hand rub (also referred to as alcohol-based hand antiseptic or alcohol rub) should be available outside of patient exam rooms, in the waiting room, and in other patient care areas when access to a sink is not readily available. Hand hygiene should be performed after every patient encounter. Hand hygiene: first and last.

Waiting Rooms

Waiting rooms and reception areas offer potential for patient-to-patient transmission of infectious agents and should be designed and maintained to minimize the risk of transmission of infectious organisms from person to person (Carrico, 2009, p. 56-2). Sufficient space to avoid overcrowding when bottlenecks occur due to overlap of appointments should be a consideration of the overall design of patient and family waiting areas.

General Housekeeping Principles

According to outpatient office infection control standards developed by the American Academy of Pediatrics (2007) all areas in the facility should be cleaned on a regular basis. Linoleum and sealed wood floors are preferred surfaces because they can be cleaned easily. Examination rooms and frequently used equipment such as bandage scissors, ultrasound probes contacting skin and ECG machines, should be cleaned daily, according to the manufacturer's recommendations (AAP Committee on Infectious Diseases, 2007, p. 660; The College of Physicians and Surgeons of Ontario, 2004). Disposable paper covers should be used in the examination rooms to cover examination tables. Waiting rooms and examination room surfaces should be cleaned with a detergent and low-level disinfectant such as a disinfectant-grade quaternary ammonium compound "registered" by the Environmental Protection Agency (EPA). (AAP Committee on Infectious Diseases, 2007). The 3M™ HB Quat Disinfectant Cleaner Concentrate is an example of this type of disinfectant.

The AAP Committee on Infectious Diseases (2007) recommends the use of disposable supplies whenever feasible. Such equipment should be used once and properly disposed of in a waste receptacle. In instances where reusable equipment is utilized, the level of disinfection or sterilization is based on whether such equipment came in direct contact with damaged or nonintact skin, body fluids, or mucous membranes. The following should be taken into consideration with regard to commonly used personal and diagnostic equipment:

1. Stethoscopes can be contaminated with antibiotic resistant organisms such as methicillin resistant staphylococcus aureus (MRSA), vancomycin-resistant *Enterococcus* species (VRE), and viral agents (AAP Committee on Infectious Diseases, 2007; BCCDC, 2004). They should be routinely disinfected between each patient use (Waghorn et al., 2005). Either a 70% isopropyl alcohol wipe or an EPA-approved disinfectant wipe labeled to be effective against hepatitis B is recommended (AAP Committee on Infectious Diseases, 2007).
2. The handle and body of otoscopes and ophthalmoscopes should be treated in the same manner as stethoscopes (AAP Committee on Infectious Diseases, 2007).

3. Blood pressure cuffs should not be placed on nonintact skin.
4. Ensure availability of plastic covers for electronic thermometers.

It is important to note that office equipment such as computer keyboards, writing implements, and patient charts can also be contaminated with infectious organisms. Although it is recommended that these items also be routinely cleaned, this is not often the case in actual practice. Diligent hand hygiene, before and after patient contact, is needed to reduce the likelihood of transfer of an infectious agent from office equipment to a patient (Carrico, 2009).

Disinfection and Sterilization

The use of surgical and medical instruments is inherent to patient care in most health care settings, including the outpatient office. Because all instruments do not require sterilization, health care practitioners must distinguish the level of cleaning that is required for various instruments to prevent the transmission of infectious organism.

Cleaning is the removal of visible soil (e.g., organic and inorganic materials) from objects and surfaces and is normally accomplished manually or mechanically using water with detergents of enzymatic products. Thorough cleaning is essential before high-level disinfection and sterilization because inorganic and organic materials that remain on the surfaces of instruments interfere with the effectiveness of these processes (Rutala, Weber, & the Healthcare Infection Control Practices Advisory Committee [HICPAC], 2008, p. 9).

Disinfection describes a process that eliminates many or all pathogenic microorganisms, except bacterial spores on inanimate objects (Rutala et al., 2008, p. 8).

Sterilization describes a process that destroys or eliminates all forms of microbial life and is carried out in health care facilities by physical or chemical methods (Rutala et al., 2008, p. 8).

Spaulding developed a classification system to determine the level of processing based on the instrument's contact with skin or tissue (Rutala, 1996). An overview of this classification system and examples of types of equipment in each category are outlined in Table 5.3 (also see Chapter 6, "Safe Patient Handling and Movement").

For office practices that perform surgical, endoscopic, or other types of invasive procedures, written policies outlining proper cleaning procedures must be developed and routinely reviewed. HCWs must have thorough knowledge of the CDC guidelines for disinfection and sterilization to prevent the spread of infectious organisms in health care facilities (see Rutala et al., 2008).

Staff responsible for the care and maintenance of this equipment must be properly trained, and ongoing education should occur to keep abreast of updated requirements and best practices.

Waste Disposal

HCP offices generate two types of waste: regulated medical waste (RMW) and municipal solid waste, commonly know as general waste (see Chapter 11, "Medical Waste Disposal").

TABLE **5.3**

Spaulding Classification of Level of Processing

CLASSIFICATION	TISSUE CONTACT	PROCESSING	EQUIPMENT
Critical	Instrument contacts sterile body tissue or the vascular system	Cleaning, then sterilization	Surgical instruments Suturing supplies Vascular catheters
Semicritical	Instrument contacts mucus membranes or nonintact skin	Cleaning, then high-level disinfection	Specula Respiratory equipment
Noncritical	Instrument only in contact with intact skin, but not mucus membranes	Cleaning, then low-level disinfection	Blood pressure cuffs Stethoscope Ophthalmoscope

Adapted from *Infection Control in the Physician's Office*, 3rd ed., by The College of Physicians and Surgeons of Ontario, 2004.

There is a lack of standardization for the definition of RMW between federal and state agencies. The term *infectious waste* is often used to describe waste that is capable of producing an infectious disease (Carrico, 2009, p. 102-2). The main categories of waste that fall under this category include sharps, cultures, POCT equipment after use, blood, blood products, and isolation waste. Regulatory bodies such as the EPA, OSHA, and other specific state agencies dictate the handling and disposal of infectious waste. It is imperative that the HCP office staff is aware of these regulations to ensure that the waste generated from the facility is disposed of properly. Staff should be provided initial and ongoing education related to identification of the different types of waste, proper handling, segregation, packaging, storage, tracking requirements, and the disposal of waste. If the decision is made to outsource this service to a contracted vendor, the vendor must be certified by the appropriate regulatory agencies for this type of waste disposal.

General waste encompasses waste produced by the office outside of the categories listed in RMW. This waste does not pose hazards to humans and the environment and is typically managed by a local government authority. See Table 5.4 for general principles for safe general waste disposal.

MINIMIZING EXPOSURE TO CONTAGIOUS ORGANISMS

The purpose of the OSHA (2008) bloodborne pathogen standard (see Chapter 2, "Bloodborne Pathogen Standard") is to protect health care workers from potential exposures to bloodborne and other potentially infectious pathogens.

TABLE 5.4

General Principles for Safe General Waste Disposal

- Use waterproof garbage containers with tight-fitting lids and foot pedal operation.
- Use impervious plastic bags to line the containers. Ensure strength of plastic bag strong enough to withstand content inside to prevent breakage.
- Do not overfill plastic bags or garbage containers
- Do not place RMW or heavy objects into plastic bags.

Adapted from *Infection Control in the Physician's Office*, 3rd ed., by The College of Physicians and Surgeons of Ontario, 2004.

In addition to defining bloodborne pathogens, OSHA mandates what employers/health care facilities must do to protect their workers from contact with potentially infectious materials. Table 5.5 outlines the major elements of the standard.

Exposure Control Plan

Prevention is the primary mechanism to thwart occupational bloodborne pathogen exposure. In addition to day-to-day best practice with regard to hand hygiene and following standard infection control precautions, HCWs should consider obtaining immunization to protect against certain common vaccine-preventable diseases, such as influenza and hepatitis B, if not already mandated to do so by institution-specific requirements. Minimally, HCWs should be aware of their immunization status. OSHA requires employers to offer the hepatitis B vaccine free of charge to newly employed staff within 10 days of hire.

A special article by Bolyard and colleages (1998) contains information covering immunization recommendations for HCWs (including paid and unpaid persons working in health care settings), recommended work restrictions for those exposed to infectious diseases, and special populations (emergency response workers, individuals who are pregnant, and personnel commonly linked to bacteria outbreaks and latex hypersensitivity).

In addition to OSHA bloodborne pathogen standards, office policies must also incorporate the CDC's current guidelines for isolation precautions (Siegel et al., 2007). Health care provider offices fall under the category of nonacute ambulatory care.

While prevention of disease transmission can be challenging in the OP office setting, development of appropriate policies and procedures to institute and maintain best infection control and prevention practices into the daily work routine are effective methods to protect both patients and HCWs from exposure.

The CDC (2005a) has additional resources for protecting HCWs.

TABLE 5.5

OSHA Blood Borne Pathogen Standard

1	Establish an exposure control plan.	Written plan to minimize or eliminate exposure. Plan must be updated annually. Annually document that consideration has been made to implement safer medical devices. Input should be sought from front line workers to identify and evaluate engineering controls.
2	Use engineering controls (isolate or remove hazard).	Include sharps disposal containers, sharp-injury protection devices, barrier devices, and needleless systems, where appropriate.
3	Enforce work practice controls.	Ensure initial and ongoing education for hand washing, sharps disposal, and lab specimen handling.
4	Provide personal protective equipment.	Employers must provide gloves, gowns, and masks as appropriate and replace as needed.
5	Provide hepatitis B vaccinations.	Provided free of charge within 10 days of hire.
6	Provide post-exposure follow-up following needlestick injuries.	Provided at no cost to the HCW.
7	Post labels and signs to indicate hazards.	Placed on containers of RMW, any container used to store infectious materials and restricted areas, as appropriate.
8	Provide training to employees.	Initially and minimally on an annual basis to review prevention, dangers, and post-exposure procedures.
9	Recordkeeping.	Must be confidential. Hepatitis B vaccination status. Training records.

Adapted from *Bloodborne Pathogen OSHA Fact Sheet*, by Occupational Safety and Health Administration, (2002).

Hand Hygiene Practice

Promotion of good hand hygiene is based on the availability and accessibility of appropriate hand hygiene agents such as soap, water, and alcohol-based hand rubs.

Table 5.6 outlines current WHO Guidelines on Hand Hygiene in Healthcare (2009b).

In addition, hand washing with soap and water is preferred after exposure to potential spore-forming pathogens including *Clostridium difficile* (WHO, 2009b) or *B. anthracis* (Carrico, 2009).

Gloves

Glove use does not replace the need for proper hand hygiene. Gloves should be located in patient exam rooms and POCT areas and are recommended in

TABLE 5.6

WHO Guidelines on Hand Hygiene in Health Care

HAND HYGIENE AGENTS	INDICATIONS
Plain lotion soap and warm water (Carrico, 2009)	Visibly dirty hands Hands visibly soiled with body fluids After using the toilet
Alcohol-based hand rubs	Preferred if hands are not visibly soiled Before and after touching a patient Before handling an invasive device for patient care After contact with body fluids and excretions, mucous membranes, nonintact skin, or wound dressings Between contact with a contaminated body site to another site on the same patient After contact with inanimate surfaces and objects After removing sterile and nonsterile gloves

From WHO, (2009).

situations in which blood or other potentially infectious material contamination is likely. In all circumstances, gloves should always be removed after caring for a patient before leaving the examination room, and they should never be reused or washed. Immediately after removing gloves, hands should be washed as close to the care area as possible.

Post-Exposure Treatment

The U.S. Public Health Service provides comprehensive guidelines for treatment of individuals exposed to certain bloodborne pathogens such as HIV and certain forms of hepatitis. The guidelines for HIV post-exposure prophylaxis were first published in 1996 with the most recent update in 2005. These guidelines review antiretroviral agents, discuss the timing of the therapy, recommendations for selection of drugs (including administration during pregnancy and emergency department physicians' knowledge of current treatment regimens), and monitoring re-evaluation of therapy (CDC, 2005b).

The most recent U.S. Public Health Service guidelines for post-exposure prophylaxis for hepatitis were last updated in 2001. This report includes risk of exposure to hepatitis B and C, hepatitis B vaccine administration, post-exposure treatment, and management (CDC, 2001). This

Staff Education

During orientation, newly hired staff should receive education regarding infection prevention and control measures, including safety devices to prevent the transmission of bloodborne pathogens. Ongoing education and competency validation is needed to ensure that staff understands the importance of their role in preventing the transmission of infection through best practice. Professional staff should keep themselves current with infection control practices and should be role models for unlicensed-assistive personnel. A nonhostile environment should be created where all members of the health care team are comfortable reminding staff and patients when lapses of infection control measures occur.

Triaging of Patients

Appropriate triage of potentially infectious patients should begin prior to their visit and continue as the patient enters the reception area.

Following is a sample of triage questions from BCCDC (2004).

Is the patient experiencing any of the following symptoms?

1. Fever or has had a fever in the last 24 hours
2. Generalized muscle aches or chills
3. Severe fatigue or generally feeling unwell
4. Severe headache (worse than usual)
5. New or worsening cough
6. Shortness of breath (worse than is normal for the patient)
7. Travel or contact with a sick person that has traveled in the last 14 days

If symptoms suggest a communicable disease, escort the patient to the exam room as soon as possible. Consider having a suspected infectious patient enter from a separate entrance to bypass the waiting room and go directly to a private exam room, or offer appointments when there is less traffic in the waiting area (e.g., early morning appointments). In addition to alcohol-based hand rubs, both tissues and no-touch receptacles for used tissue disposal should be conveniently located and consistently available in patient waiting areas. In general, avoidance of crowding and shortened wait times in reception/waiting areas is recommended.

Point of Care Testing

Once the patient has been examined, one of the methods to assist in the proper diagnosis and treatment of an infectious disease is point of care testing (POCT). POCT is defined as testing at or near the site of patient care (Esposito, 2008). One of the advantages of POCT is it provides the HCP with results in a timely manner. POCT performed in health care provider offices are regulated under the Clinical Laboratory Improvement Amendments (CLIA) law passed by Congress. These amendments outline requirements that offices must meet in order to perform tests on human specimens. If POCT is to be performed in a HCP's office, the office must be licensed. A "Certificate of Waiver" license is required by an office that only performs waited tests. The National Academy of Clinical Biochemistry has developed EBP guidelines for infectious disease POCT (Campbell et al., 2006). These guidelines will assist HCPs in the decision to utilize a specific POCT based on levels of evidence and national recommendations. Web sites of interest for more information related to POCT are located in Table 5.7.

TABLE 5.7

Point of Care Testing Web Sites

TOPIC	LINK
CLIA overview	http://www.cms.hhs.gov/CLIA/01_Overview.asp#TopOfPage
List of waived test	http://www.cms.hhs.gov/CLIA/10_Categorization_of_Tests.asp#TopOfPage
Evidenced-based practice guidelines for POCT	http://www.ngc.gov/summary/summary.aspx?ss=15&doc_id=10818&nbr=005643&string=

HCP offices are not routinely inspected by regulatory agencies such as the Department of Health (DOH) or the College of American Pathologists (CAP), but are inspected by OSHA under the federal clause related to the bloodborne pathogen standard (Esposito, 2008).

Multiple factors are required to render accurate results, but a review of two statistical terms assists the provider in selecting a valid and reliable testing kit. The decision to use POCT also requires knowledge of the accuracy of specific tests used in the office setting (see Chapter 13, "Methods of Surveillance"). *Sensitivity* and *specificity* are statistical terms that are applied to a wide variety of clinical diagnostic tests ranging from radiographic and diagnostic imaging to those conducted in the laboratory. Sensitivity refers to the number of times a test yields true positive results, while specificity indicates the number of times a test yields true negative results (American Academy of Family Physicians [AAFP], 2009). Both, of course, are important for the clinician to know because such results will guide diagnosis and treatment. The closer a test is to 100% sensitivity or specificity, the greater the accuracy for either a true positive or a true negative, respectively.

In the following example, a patient comes into the office with a sore throat and receives a POCT such as a rapid streptococcal test. The patient will have either a negative or positive result. A throat culture is also obtained, which is sent to the laboratory. Table 5.8 demonstrates the four scenarios that might occur.

TABLE 5.8

Sensitivity and Specificity Scenarios

	LAB CULTURE POSITIVE	LAB CULTURE NEGATIVE
Rapid Streptococcal Test positive	True positive	False positive
Rapid Streptococcal Test negative	False negative	True negative

Examples of Commercially Available POCTs

Upper respiratory symptoms can be caused by allergens, viruses, bacteria, and other infectious organisms. Prompt recognition and treatment of influenza can reduce the severity of symptoms and reduce the virus from replicating. In order to rapidly confirm a diagnosis of influenza, a CLIA waived influenza A + B POCT can be utilized. This test can aid in the diagnosis by detecting both A and B viral antigens in about 10–15 minutes. The nasal swab technique yields the following accuracy rates:

Sensitivity: A 94%, B 70%—Nasal Swab

Specificity: A 90%, B 97%—Nasal Swab (Quidel Corporation, 2008)

There are several POCTs to identify streptococcal bacteria (Group A), a common cause of pharyngitis or throat infections. This aids the practitioner in differentiating bacterial from viral mediated pharyngitis to ensure proper treatment. Most rapid strep tests have a sensitivity of 95% and a specificity as high as 98%. Review individual testing kits for their sensitivity and specificity percentages (MedicineNet, n.d.).

Whichever tests or commercial kits are selected for office use, the manufacturer's guidelines must be strictly adhered to for performance of the test, interpretation of test results, quality control, and storage. It is imperative that staff that is responsible for POCT is properly trained and that their competency is revalidated on an ongoing basis.

Patient Education

Once the patient is diagnosed with an infectious disease, education is encouraged to ensure that the patient and family members understand their role in reducing the spread of infection. Information should include average length of communicability, prevention of spread of the disease in the household or to others, instructions for medications or treatments dispensed, further follow-up, and methods to prevent future outbreaks. The HCP must give accurate, up-to-date information, validate patient understanding of the education, dispel myths, and provide reassurance.

Part of the overall strategy in the prevention of transmission of organisms is the promotion of hand hygiene. The CDC encourages partnering with patients to promote hand hygiene and covering the mouth and nose when coughing occurs. The CDC Web site offers a multitude of resources free of charge to promote health hygiene in the community specific to minimizing transmission of infection. Patient education can be facilitated through use of signage and other educational materials placed in strategic locations in both waiting areas and treatment rooms. For an example of educational materials that are available, see http://www.cdc.gov/flu/protect/pdf/covercough_hcp8-5x11.pdf. During times of the year when the incidence of respiratory illness in the community is high, the CDC (2009) further recommends offering masks to persons who are coughing. Such individuals are encouraged to remain at least 3 feet from others when in common waiting areas. Such practices may be instituted year-round according to facility-specific policy.

Antibiotic-Resistant Organisms

Antimicrobials have wide-scale use in humans, animals, and agriculture. As a result, organisms have mutated and developed resistance to commonly pre-scribed antibiotics, and effective treatment is a growing challenge to HCPs worldwide (see Chapter 16, "Antibiotic-Resistant Infections"). Between 5% and 10% of all hospital patients in the United States develop a hospital-acquired infection at a cost of more than $5 billion annually (National Institute of Allergy and Infectious Diseases, 2009).

Resistant organisms can be a part of a patient's normal flora for an extended period of time. These organisms include MRSA, VRE, and extended-spectrum B-lactamase—producing or multiply-resistant Gram-negative bacteria. The usual route of transmission of antibiotic-resistant organisms is by the hands of health care personnel (Carrico, 2009, p. 56-5). Hand hygiene is a must, particularly in this population of patient. These known antibiotic-resistant patients should have alerts placed in their medical record to aid in the appropriate infection control measures occurring on subsequent visits.

Community Outbreaks

Over the past decade, there has been an alarming rise in the number of serious community-acquired infections, including MRSA, severe acute respiratory syn-drome (SARS), HIN1 flu, and others (MedicineNet, 2008; WHO, 2009a). It has been known for decades that improved control of spread of infection can often be managed if appropriate infection control guidelines are adhered to by both HCPs and members of the community at large.

A wide variety of resources containing information for both HCWs and com-munity members is available via the Internet or from government agencies such as the CDC, the Veteran's Administration, or state and local Departments of Health. Resources typically include toolkits, posters, or flyers; patient and family handouts, and multimedia products. These tools are often free of charge and provide up-to-date information and standards on ways to prevent or minimize risk of exposure to contagious disease and bloodborne pathogens. In addition, materials are often available in various languages to meet the needs of English as Second Language (ESL) populations.

Maintaining a current list of resources and Internet addresses in the office setting is one way to ensure access to current standards and patient education information on topics of interest with regard to community outbreaks and rec-ommended control measures.

Table 5.9 provides Web sites that provide up-to-date information for health care professionals, patients, families, and other interested members of the com-munity about communicable and contagious diseases often encountered in the community. It is imperative that patients and health care professionals continue to keep themselves up-to-date with the rapidly changing standards, evaluation, and treatment of infectious diseases.

TABLE 5.9

Web Sites for Information about Communicable and Contagious Diseases

ASSOCIATION	WEB SITE	COMMENT
Association for Professionals in Infection Control and Epidemiology (APIC)	www.apic.org/AM/ Template.cfm?Section= Practice&Template=/CM/ HTMLDisplay.cfm& ContentID=11355& MicrositeID=0&Website Key=28980e36-1554- 46a7-8e91-d7f06abd0a11	This Web site provides information to HCWs and their role in the prevention of influenza.
Centers For Disease Control	www.cdc.gov	This Web site has information for HCPs for: ■ Respiratory hygiene/cough etiquette in a health care setting (www.cdc.gov/flu/professionals/ infectioncontrol/resphygiene.htm); printable educational poster to post in waiting and examination rooms for a reminder to covering your cough. There are versions available in multiple languages (www.cdc.gov/flu/ protect/covercough.htm). ■ Influenza and surveillance activity in the United States (www.cdc.gov/flu/ weekly/fluactivity.htm). ■ General information, symptoms, diagnosis, treatment, questions and answers related to the H1N1 (Swine) flu (www.cdc.gov/h1n1flu/general_ info.htm). ■ Overview, prevention, control and, education material related to community-associated methicillin-resistant *Staphylococcus aureus* (CA-MRSA) (www.cdc.gov/ncidod/ dhqp/ar_mrsa_ca.html). ■ Topics related to infection control in health care settings (www.cdc.gov/ ncidod/dhqp/index.html). ■ Overview of Severe Acute Respiratory Syndrome (SARS); reviews the 2003 outbreak, symptoms, how SARS is spread, diagnosis, and information for travelers (www.cdc.gov/ncidod/sars/ factsheet.htm).

(Continued)

TABLE 5.9

(Continued)

ASSOCIATION	WEB SITE	COMMENT
U.S. Government Flu Information Web Site	www.flu.gov	This Web site has information for individuals and families to know what to do about influenza, vaccination, prevention, and treatment. There is information for professionals to assist in planning for outbreaks.
Association of Professionals in Infection Control and Epidemiology (APIC)	www.preventinfection.org	Informative Web site for consumers for prevention of infection.
	www.preventinfection. org//AM/Template. cfm?Section=Home	A partnership with national organizations has educational materials for health care consumers on ways to protect themselves against health care–associated infections.
Veteran's Administration's (VA)	www.publichealth.va.gov/ healthinfo.asp	This Web site has infectious disease information for veterans, the public, and health professionals.
Veteran's Administration's (VA)	www.publichealth.va.gov/ infectiondontpassiton/ index.asp	This Web site has information on prevention of the spread of infectious organisms.
State Department of Health (as an example, New Jersey)	www.state.nj.us/health	Discusses local issues of community outbreaks and resources in the state.
World Health Organization (WHO)	www.who.int/csr/ disease/swineflu/en	This Web site can be utilized for global pandemic (H1N1) alerts and responses.

Partnering with the community provides the cornerstone to control the spread of these and other infections. Core components of a partnership model include:

1. Identification of at-risk individuals and populations
2. Communication of vital information and facts
3. Educational strategies that are proven to be effective for various learner groups
4. Role-modeling by health care workers to the community related to best practices and behaviors to prevent the spread of infection

POST-TEST QUESTIONS

5-1. Which of the following does NOT need to be disinfected or sterilized?
  a. Stethoscope
  b. Otoscope handle
  c. Computer keyboards
  d. Disposable thermometer

5-2. The process that destroys or eliminates all forms of microbial life and is carried out in health care facilities by physical or chemical methods is called:
  a. Cleaning
  b. High-level disinfection
  c. Low-level disinfection
  d. Sterilization

5-3. Which of the following is considered general waste or municipal waste?
  a. Sharps
  b. Soiled tissue
  c. Blood products
  d. Isolation waste

5-4. OSHA requires employers to offer which of the following vaccines to newly employed staff?
  a. Hepatitis A
  b. Hepatitis B
  c. Varicella zoster
  d. Meningococcal

5-5. An exposure control plan is a plan to:
  a. Minimize or eliminate exposure to bloodborne pathogens
  b. Describes the treatment necessary following a needlestick injury
  c. Should be updated every 3 to 5 years
  d. Should be distributed to all patients annually

References

American Academy of Family Physicians. (2009). *Sensitivity and specificity.* Retrieved December 24, 2009, from http://www.aafp.org/online/en/home/publications/journals/afp/ebm toolkit/ebmglossary/afppoems.html#Parsys73206

American Academy of Pediatrics Committee on Infectious Diseases. (2007). Infection prevention and control in pediatric ambulatory settings. *Pediatrics, 120,* 650–665.

BC Centre for Disease Control. (2004). *Guidelines for infection prevention and control in the physician's offices.* Retrieved August 16, 2010 from http://www.bccdc.ca/NR/rdonlyres/84DA413D-C943-4B5F-94F1-794C5B76C9CE/0/InfectionControl_GF_IC_Physician_Office.pdf

Bolyard, R.A., Tablan, O.C., Williams, W.W., Pearson, M.L., Shaprio, C.N., & Deitchman, S. D. (1998). *Guidelines for infection control in health care personnel.* Retrieved December 28, 2009, from http://www.cdc.gov/ncidod/dhqp/pdf/guidelines/InfectControl98.pdf

Campbell, S., Campos, J., Hall, G.S., LeBar, W.D., Greene, W., Roush, D., et al. (2006). Infectious disease. In National Academy of Clinical Biochemistry (Ed.), *Laboratory medicine practice guidelines: Evidence-based practice for point-of-care testing* (pp. 76–94). Washington, DC: National Academy of Clinical Biochemistry. Retrieved December 22, 2009, from http://www.ngc.gov/summary/summary.aspx?ss=15&doc_id=10818&nbr=005643&string

Carrico, R. (Ed.). (2009). *APIC text of infection control and epidemiology* (3rd ed., Vols. I & II). Washington, DC: Association for Professionals in Infection Control and Epidemiology, Inc.

Centers for Disease Control and Prevention. (2001). *Updated U.S. public health service guidelines for the management of occupational exposures to HBV, HCV, and HIV and recommendations for postexposure prophylaxis*. Retrieved December 28, 2009, from http://www.cdc.gov/mmwr/PDF/rr/rr5011.pdf

Centers for Disease Control and Prevention. (2005a). *Protecting healthcare personnel*. Retrieved December 28, 2009, from http://www.cdc.gov/ncidod/dhqp/worker.html

Centers for Disease Control and Prevention. (2005b). *Updated U.S. public health service guidelines for the management of occupational exposures to HIV and recommendations for postexposure prophylaxis*. Retrieved December 28, 2009, from http://www.cdc.gov/mmwr/preview/mmwrhtml/rr5409a1.htm

Centers for Disease Control and Prevention. (2009). *Respiratory hygiene/cough etiquette in healthcare setting*. Retrieved December 28, 2009, from http://www.cdc.gov/flu/professionals/infectioncontrol/resphygiene.htm

Esposito, E. (2008). Point of care testing. *AAACN Viewpoint, 30*(6), 1.

MedicineNet. (2003) *The SARS epidemic in perspective*. Retrieved August 16, 2010, from http://www.medicinenet.com/script/main/art.asp?articlekey=23593

MedicineNet. (2008). *New infectious diseases on the rise*. Retrieved December 26, 2009, from http://www.medicinenet.com/script/main/art.asp?articlekey=87334

National Institute of Allergy and Infectious Diseases. (2009). *Antimicrobial (drug) resistance quick facts*. Retrieved on December 21, 2009, from http://www3.niaid.nih.gov/topics/antimicrobialResistance/Understanding/quickFacts.htm

Occupational Safety and Health Administration. (2002). *Bloodborne pathogen OSHA fact sheet*. Retrieved December 21, 2009, from http://www.osha.gov/OshDoc/data_BloodborneFacts/bbfact01.pdf

Occupational Safety and Health Administration. (2008). *Bloodborne pathogens—1910–1030*. Retrieved December 28, 2009, from http://www.osha.gov/pls/oshaweb/owadisp.show_document?p_table=STANDARDS&p_id=10051

Pyrek, Kelly. (2002). Preventing infections in the ambulatory surgery setting. *Infection Control Today*. Retrieved November 10, 2009, from http://www.infectioncontroltoday.com/articles/403/403_281feat3.html

Quidel Corporation. (2008). *QuickVue influenza test product specifications*. Retrieved November 23, 2009, from http://www.quidel.com/products/product_detail.php?prod=56&group=1&show=spec

Rutala, W. A. (1996). *APIC guideline for selection and use of disinfectants*. Retrieved August 16, 2010, from: http://www.inicc.org/guias/16_gddisinfAJIC-96.pdf

Rutala, W.A., Weber, D.J., & the Healthcare Infection Control Practices Advisory Committee (HICPAC). (2008). *Guideline for disinfection and sterilization in healthcare facilities*. Retrieved November 23, 2009, from http://www.cdc.gov/ncidod/dhqp/pdf/guidelines/Disinfection_Nov_2008.pdf

Siegel, J.D., Rhinehart, E., Jackson, M., Chiarello, L., & the Healthcare Infection Control Practices Advisory Committee (HICPAC). (2007). *Guideline for isolation precautions: Preventing transmission of infectious agents in healthcare settings*. Retrieved November 23, 2009, from http://www.cdc.gov/ncidod/dhqp/pdf/guidelines/Isolation2007.pdf

The College of Physicians and Surgeons of Ontario. (2004). *Infection control in the physician's office* (3rd ed.). Retrieved November 11, 2009, from http://www.cpso.on.ca/uploadedFiles/policies/guidelines/office/Infection_Controlv2.pdf

The Facility Guidelines Institute, The American Institute of Architects Academy of Architecture for Health with the assistance from the U.S. Department of Health and Human Services. (2006). *Guidelines for design and construction of healthcare facilities*. Washington, DC: American Institute of Architects.

Waghorn, D.J., Wan, W.Y., Greaves, C., Whittome, N., Bosley, H.C., & Cantrill, S. (2005). Stethoscopes: A study of contamination and the effectiveness of disinfection procedures. *British Journal of Infection Control, 6,* 15–17.

World Health Organization. (2009a). *Infection prevention and control during health care for con-firmed, probable, or suspected cases of pandemic (H1N1) 2009 virus infection and influenza like illnesses.* Retrieved December 26, 2009, from http://www.who.int/csr/resources/publi cations/cp150_2009_1612_ipc_interim_guidance_h1n1.pdf

World Health Organization. (2009b). *WHO guidelines on hand hygiene in health care.* Retrieved November 11, 2009, from http://whqlibdoc.who.int/publications/2009/9789241597906_ eng.pdf

Web Sites

http://www.cdc.gov
http://www.cdc.gov/ncidod/dhqp/index.html
http://www.cms.hhs.gov/CLIA/10_Categorization_of_Tests.asp#TopOfPage
http://www.cms.hhs.gov/CLIA/01_Overview.asp#TopOfPage
http://www.cpso.on.ca/uploadedFiles/policies/guidelines/office/Infection_Controlv2.pdf
http://www.osha.gov
http://www.osha.gov/OshDoc/data_BloodborneFacts/bbfact01.pdf
http://www.who.int/en/

Safe Patient Handling and Movement

6

This chapter includes topics on the types of and disinfection of safe patient handling equipment. The cleaning of the different types of equipment are reviewed. The content differentiates between the use of disposable and nondisposable or washable equipment. Disinfection procedures for equipment are reviewed. Finally, the use of germicidal agents and the Centers for Disease Control and Prevention (CDC) guidelines for the steps in the laundry process are discussed.

OBJECTIVES

1. Identify a reliable resource of authority for infection control guidelines.
2. Recognize which aspects of environmental control guidelines are relevant to safe patient handling equipment and accessories.
3. Identify the factors influencing the disinfection procedures for environmental surfaces, i.e. medical equipment.
4. Describe methods to clean and disinfect safe patient handling hardware.
5. Describe methods to clean and disinfect safe patient handling accessories.

PRE-TEST QUESTIONS

6-1. What authority establishes guidelines for infection control standards in hospitals and other health care settings?
   a. The Local Board of Health
   b. The facility's environmental services/housekeeping department manager
   c. The clinical team taking care of the patient
   d. The Centers for Disease Control and Prevention
   e. a and d

6-2. Which aspects of health care environmental control guidelines affect safe patient handling equipment (hardware) and accessories (slings, "software")?
   a. Air and water guidelines
   b. Environmental services and laundry/bedding guidelines
   c. Environmental sampling and animals in health care setting guidelines
   d. Regulated medical waste guidelines

6-3. Which factors influence the choice of disinfection procedure for environmental surfaces?
   a. The nature of the item to be disinfected
   b. The number of microorganisms present and the amount of organic soil present
   c. The resistance of the microorganisms to the inactivating effects of the germicide used
   d. Type and concentration of germicide used and duration and temperature of germicide contact
   e. All of the above

6-4. What steps are correct in the recommended process for cleaning safe patient handling hardware?
   a. Hand-washing awareness campaign
   b. Clean surfaces of debris and soil
   c. Disinfect surfaces with recommended strength and type of disinfectant
   d. Heat sterilize the surfaces
   e. b and c

6-5. What steps are correct in recommended process for cleaning safe patient handling software (e.g., slings and accessories)?
   a. Removal of used accessory from area where it was used or contaminated
   b. Containment and transport of the used/contaminated accessory
   c. Antimicrobial action of the laundering process
   d. Transport, distribution, and storage of cleaned accessories
   e. All of the above

Health care workers (HCWs) are at risk for infection daily while at work. Medical equipment can become contaminated with infectious materials, which means health care workers who come in contact with the contaminated object can be infected and/or contribute to cross contamination and hospital acquired infection(s). Therefore, health care facilities must have policies and procedures in place for the soiled and contaminated items.

Such inherent conditions create an environment in which a number of varying microorganisms can exist and health care–associated infections (HAIs) can occur. Therefore, whenever health care facilities introduce new equipment to their inventory, they must plan for its cleaning. In fact, it is worthwhile for facilities to consider or evaluate a potential device's environmental management requirements prior to purchase so that devices can be selected that allow the facility to meet the maintenance requirements without undue hardship. (See the CDC's 2008 Guidelines for the Disinfection and Sterilization in Healthcare Facilities.)

One specific type of equipment commonly found in many health care settings is safe patient handling and movement (SPHM) equipment. Utilizing such equipment reduces the risk of staff musculoskeletal injuries and promotes a safer work environment for staff and patients (Waters, 2007). Infection control practices regarding SPHM are discussed in the *Guidelines for Environmental Infection Control in Healthcare Facilities* (Sehulster et al., 2004).

SAFE PATIENT HANDLING TECHNOLOGY

SPHM technology can be thought of as loosely divided into two main categories. One category is hardware, which comprises such items as overhead hoists, floor based hoists, slide boards, powered canisters that work with inflatable products, and externally attached powered transport products (see Figures 6.1–6.3). Such hardware surfaces are usually nonporous and can include plastic, aluminum, steel, rubber, and composite .

The other category of safe patient handling technology is software, which comprises such items as fabric slings, antifriction sheets and surfaces, and inflatable surfaces (see Figures 6.4–6.6). These software surfaces are usually porous and can include polyester, nylon, cotton, and blended synthetic materials.

Development of new safe patient handling technology is ongoing, therefore, please consult with and follow the manufacturer's cleaning guidelines, development of new safe patient handling technology is ongoing, therefore, please consult with and follow the manufacturer's cleaning guidelines.

FIGURE 6.1

Close-up of overhead hoist on rail, Guldmann ™

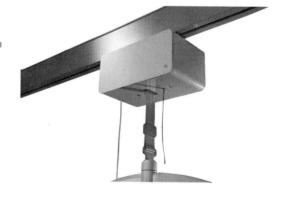

FIGURE 6.2

Floor-based hoist, Guldmann ™

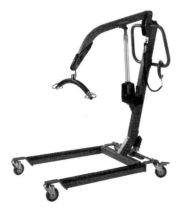

FIGURE 6.3

Lateral slide board

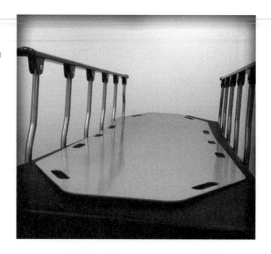

FIGURE 6.4

Sling, Guldmann ™

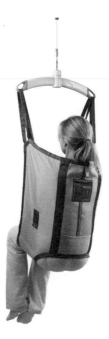

Additionally, awareness of the surface and material composition\of any purchased technology, will assist in determining the appropriate cleaning procedures. The hardware category of SPHM technology falls into the CDC guidelines for environmental surfaces of medical equipment; while the software category falls into the CDC guidelines for laundry and bedding (Sehulster et al., 2004).

Hardware: Medical Equipment

To successfully clean hardware surfaces, two steps are used: (1) cleaning, followed by (2) terminal processing or disinfecting. There are several factors that affect the choice of disinfection:

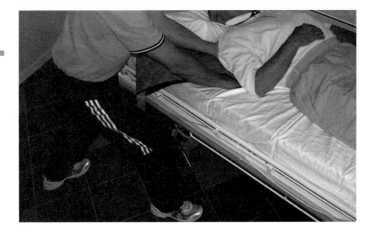

FIGURE 6.5

Antifriction sheet

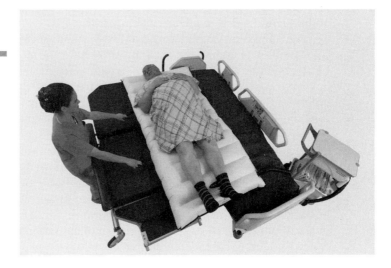

FIGURE 6.6

Power inflate lateral transfer device

Courtesy of Smart Medical Technology, Inc.

1. The nature of the item to be disinfected
2. The number of microorganisms present
3. The amount of organic soil present
4. The resistance of the microorganisms to the inactivating effects of the germicide used
5. The type and concentration of germicide used
6. The duration and temperature of germicide contact

Standard precautions with the appropriate type of personnel protective equipment (PPE) necessary for the task should always be used when cleaning (see Chapter 2, "Bloodborne Pathogen Standard"). Surfaces must first be cleaned to remove organic matter and visible soil. Failure to first clean a surface, by physical scrubbing with detergent and surfactants then rinsing or wiping with water, can interfere with the success of the disinfection phase.

The CDC uses Spaulding's (1968) classification system, which describes three levels of germicidal activity: sterilization, high-level disinfection, and low-level disinfection. The system also classifies medical devices as critical, semicritical, or noncritical based on the safety risk associated with device contamination. The level of germicidal activity combined with the medical device classification of the item to be cleaned determines the appropriate level of disinfection for the surface.

Germicidal agents that are used for low-level disinfection are regulated by the Environmental Protection Agency (EPA) and apply to SPHM equipment. The manufacturer's directions for use (DFU) of the germicidal agent are essential and must be followed exactly for the microbial inactivation effects to occur. The DFU may include storage temperature, storage longevity, and appropriate concentration of the agent for application, as well as appropriate amount of the agent, contact temperature, and surface contact (exposure) time. Failure to abide by the usage directions could compromise the germicidal agent's effects and might not accomplish the desired disinfecting result.

For SPHM hardware items that are portable, including those that move from one care area to another or have the potential to be shared, the equipment should be cleaned and disinfected between each patient use. Special attention should be given to high touch areas, that is, surfaces of the device that have the highest potential for hand or intact skin contact and to any area of the device exposed to body fluids or substances or other organic matter. Hardware items that are permanently affixed in a particular care area and have no potential to be shared between different patients can be cleaned and disinfected after each patient discharge. Should visible soil or debris become evident during the course of a patient stay, equipment surfaces should, at a minimum, be cleaned of visible soiling.

The use of barrier protection is another option for facilities to consider, especially if the surfaces are touched frequently by gloved hands during the delivery of patient care, are likely to become contaminated with body substances, or are difficult to clean. An example of such barrier protection is a plastic wrapping. Such barriers must be changed between patients and need to be removed after use, while the caregiver is still gloved. Practicality and expense of barrier protection should be weighed in comparison to the cleaning and disinfecting requirements. An area for further consideration related to hygiene procedures is that of the use of probiotic cleaning agents. Probiotic cleaning agents are thought to break down biofilm and bad bacteria while preserving good bacteria. This is a growing field and studies examining their effects on safe patient handling technology is warranted.

Software: Slings and Antifriction Surfaces

Methods to clean and sanitize the items in the software category of SPHM equipment are guided by the CDC guidelines for management of laundry in health care facilities (Sehulster et al., 2004). Reports of HAIs linked to contaminated fabrics are very few in number, and in light of the volume of fabric and linen laundered annually in the United States (estimated to be 5 billion pounds), the existing practices used for controlling infection through laundry sources are reasonable to continue.

CDC guidelines state, "Through a combination of soil removal, pathogen removal, and pathogen inactivation, contaminated laundry can be rendered hygienically clean. Hygienically clean laundry carries negligible risk to HCWs and patients, provided that the clean textiles, fabric and clothing are not inadvertently contaminated before use."

SPHM software can be reusable or disposable (see Figure 6.7). Reusable software would follow the guidelines and procedures associated with laundry management, while the disposable or single patient use software would be discarded (Sehulster et al., 2004; see also Chapter 11, "Medical Waste Disposal").

Should reusable software have manufacturer's DFU guidelines for an alternative method of cleaning and disinfection, then those directions should be followed. Remember that the manufacturer's DFU on cleaning does not eliminate the facility's responsibility for proper cleaning and disinfection. For example, if a manufacturer's guidelines states that a software item can be surface wiped with a disinfectant cloth between patients, then the health care facility should ensure that the chemical agent in the surface wipe is a sufficient method, is of sufficient concentration, and has sufficient contact surface time to inactivate the microbes present.

There are several steps in a laundry process, each with specifications of proper procedures within the step. Cleaning the soiled items, alone, does not constitute laundry management. The manufacturer's DFU for cleaning the fabric item should

FIGURE 6.7

Disposable or single patient use sling, Guldmann ™

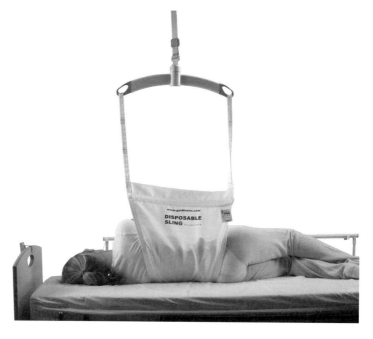

be followed according to the criteria specified. If not readily apparent, consult with the manufacturer to determine the fabric's material composition so that any unique composition can be assessed and aligned with guidelines or criteria specified by the CDC for fabric or textiles. HCWs should follow standard precautions with PPE that are appropriate to the task, similar to the procedure for cleaning SPHM hardware.

Steps in the Laundry Process

1. Remove used or contaminated item(s).
2. Contain and transport used or contaminated item(s).
3. Sort and clean used or contaminated item(s).
4. Package and distribute cleaned item(s).
5. Store clean item(s).

When removing safe patient handling software from areas where use occurred, agitation and shaking of the items should be kept to a minimum to prevent or minimize any aerosolized contaminated lint. Used items should be placed in laundry bags that will not leak and that have sufficient tensile strength for the load, and the bags must be labeled appropriately to reflect the soiled or contaminated contents.

If used software continue to be needed by the patient or staff, then the software item(s) should remain in the care area and labeled to prevent an incorrect assignment, especially in semiprivate care areas. Used software should be stored in a consistent spot, while its use continues to be required. After use is no longer needed or the item(s) become excessively soiled to warrant laundering, then the process for laundering should be followed.

Used software should be transported by cart or by a laundry chute, if available. Should surfaces on the transport carts or chutes become contaminated from direct exposure to soiled software, then such surfaces should be appropriately cleaned and disinfected.

Sorting laundry, including the SPHM software, assists in identifying any sharp or foreign objects that might injure HCWs or damage equipment. Sorting also groups like items to help in the packaging and clean distribution process. The sorting and laundering process may take place at a location that is external to the health care facility. Such external locations are sometimes part of the health care facility's corporate structure, while others are separate companies that contract and manage laundry services on behalf of the facility. It is the responsibility of the health care facility to ensure that the laundry procedures and processes meet the standards set by the relevant authorities regardless of where or by whom the services are performed.

It is during the actual laundering cycles that fabrics, textiles, and garments become free of vegetative pathogens, that is, hygienically clean, but not sterile. The interaction of the mechanical aspects of diluting the items in water and water agitation removes large quantities of microorganisms; the thermal aspects of water temperature and the chemical factors of detergent and other chemical additives produce the antimicrobial effect on fabric and SPHM soft-ware. CDC guidelines cite a minimum water temperature of 160°F (71°C) for 25 minutes for hot water washing. Although other national and international guidelines vary, sometimes citing lower water temperatures and/or less agita-tion time with reasonable results, U.S. health care facilities should follow CDC guidelines in addition to any relevant local requirements (Orr, Holliday, Jones, Robson, & Perry, 2002; Fijan, Koren, Cencic, & Sostar-Turk, 2007; Smith, Neil, Davidson, & Davidson, 1987).

Laundering Cycles

- Flush
- Main wash
- Detergent/chemical exposure
- Rinse
- Souring

It is thought that the addition of chlorine bleach (at 50–150 ppm, activated at minimum temperatures of 135°–145°F) enhances the disinfection effect (Sehul-ster et al., 2004); however, the studies examining its efficacy are few in number and not recent (Smith et al., 1987).

Considering the harsh effect chlorine bleach can have on fabrics, especially fabrics that have flame-retardant or other specialized properties, the use of chlo-rine bleach alternatives (such as oxygen-based bleach) should be explored and their efficacy studied.

The last cycles for laundering include rinsing and pH correction (sour). Rinsing assists to clear dislodged debris, microorganisms, and additives from the fabrics; pH correction, performed by adding mild acid, reduces an alkaline pH tendency that might occur via the water supply or additives. A more acidic pH for fabrics is thought to inactivate some microorganisms and reduce re-sidual alkali in the fabric, which can cause skin irritation in patients (Sehulster et al., 2004).

Following washing, fabrics and SPHM software are dried. Review and fol-low the manufacturer's guidelines for tumble drying, as there may be limits on the maximum allowable temperature exposure. Studies that have examined lower water temperature washing have found further reduction in microbes after a tumble drying phase of 93.3°C (199°F; Smith et al., 1987).

Packaging and distribution of clean textiles, fabrics, and SPHM software occurs after cleaning has been completed. Laundry facility standards specify the need for separate soiled and clean laundry areas, thereby minimizing the risk of cross contamination (Sehulster et al., 2004). Wrapping or covering clean fabrics prevents dust, debris, or contact with soiled linen if they are in close proximity during any handling or transport phases. Lastly, clean fabric and SPHM software should be stored in a manner that keeps them dry and free of any contaminants. Many health care facilities achieve this by storing laundry or SPHM software in covered carts, if they are not individually wrapped (see Figure 6.8).

FIGURE 6.8

Example facility cart for
clean storage

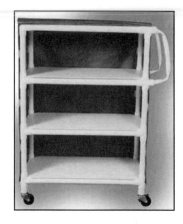

CONCLUSION

The infection control and hygienic management of today's SPHM technology—
hardware, such as hoists, and software, such as slings—is not unusual nor outside of what is available for recommended, effective methods. It is however,
important to emphasize that as health care facilities introduce this technology
into their environment, they prepare to integrate it with their facility-wide plan
of environmental care. This means that there are designated procedures, protocols, and persons and or departments responsible for the hygienic management
of this technology.

POST-TEST QUESTIONS

6-1. What authority establishes guidelines for infection control standards in
hospitals and other health care settings?
   a. The Local Board of Health
   b. The facility's environmental services/housekeeping department manager
   c. The clinical team taking care of the patient
   d. The Centers for Disease Control and Prevention
   e. a and d

6-2. Which aspects of health care environmental control guidelines affect safe
patient handling equipment (hardware) and accessories (slings, "software")?
   a. Air and water guidelines
   b. Environmental services and laundry/bedding guidelines
   c. Environmental sampling and animals in health care setting guidelines
   d. Regulated medical waste guidelines

6-3. Which factors influence the choice of disinfection procedure for environmental surfaces?
   a. The nature of the item to be disinfected
   b. The number of microorganisms present and the amount of organic soil
present

    c. The resistance of the microorganisms to the inactivating effects of the germicide used

    d. Type and concentration of germicide used and duration and temperature of germicide contact

    e. All of the above

6-4. What steps are correct in the recommended process for cleaning safe patient handling hardware?

    a. Hand-washing awareness campaign

    b. Clean surfaces of debris and soil

    c. Disinfect surfaces with recommended strength and type of disinfectant

    d. Heat sterilize the surfaces

    e. b and c

6-5. What steps are correct in recommended process for cleaning safe patient handling software (e.g., slings and accessories)?

    a. Removal of used accessory from area where it was used or contaminated

    b. Containment and transport of the used/contaminated accessory

    c. Antimicrobial action of the laundering process

    d. Transport, distribution, and storage of cleaned accessories

    e. All of the above

References

Centers for Disease Control and Prevention. Healthcare Infection Control Practices Advisory Committee (HICPAC). (2008). *Guidelines for the disinfection and sterilization in healthcare facilities.* Retrieved July 16, 2010, from http://www.cdc.gov/hicpac/Disinfection_Steriliza tion/6_0disinfection.html

Fijan, S., Koren, S., Cencic, A., & Sostar-Turk, S. (2007). Antimicrobial disinfection effect of a laundering procedure for hospital textiles against various indicator bacteria and fungi using different substrates for simulating human excrements. *Diagnl Microbiology Infectious Disease, 57*(3), 251–257.

Orr, K.E., Holliday, M.G., Jones, A.L., Robson, I., & Perry, J.D. (2002). Survival of enterococci during laundry processing. *The Journal of Hospital Infection, 50*(2), 133–139.

Sehulster, L.M., Chinn, R.Y.W., Arduino, M.J., Carpenter, J., Donlan, R., Ashford, D., et al. (2004). *Guidelines for environmental infection control in health-care facilities. Recommendations from CDC and the Healthcare Infection Control Practices Advisory Committee (HICPAC).* Chicago: American Society for Healthcare Engineering/American Hospital Association.

Smith, J.A., Neil, K.R., Davidson, C.G., Davidson, R.W. (1987). Effect of water temperature on bacterial killing in laundry. *Infection Control, 8*(5), 204–209.

Spaulding, E.H. (1968). Chemical disinfection of medical and surgical materials. In C. Lawrence & S.S. Block (Eds.), *Disinfection, sterilization, and preservation* (pp. 517–531). Philadelphia: Lea & Febiger.

Waters, T. (2007). When is it safe to manually lift a patient? *American Journal of Nursing, 107*(8), 40–45.

Web Sites

http://www.guldmann.net/Default.aspx?ID=3665

http://kingdompictures.com

http://www.master-care.dk/files/manager/hhb1engelsk2010(1).pdf

http://www.medicalproductsdirect.com/linencarts.html

7

Health Care–Associated Infections

This chapter includes topics on health care–associated infections and how the infection affects patients. Treatment options for health care–associated infections are reviewed. The content describes methods to prevent or decrease the spread of health care–associated infections. There is discussion on microorganisms commonly seen and risk factors for health care–associated infections. Finally, high-touch areas for environmental cleaning and patient psychosocial effects of infection are discussed.

OBJECTIVES

1. Define health care–associated infections.
2. List three health care–associated infections affecting patients.
3. Review treatment options for health care–associated infections.
4. Describe methods to prevent or decrease the spread of health care–associated infections.

PRE-TEST QUESTIONS

7-1. Which of the following terms refers to a hospital-acquired infection?
   a. Nosocomial
   b. Latent
   c. Smoldering
   d. Active
7-2. An organism commonly associated with health care–associated infections is:
   a. *Haemophilus influenza*
   b. *Streptococcus pneumoniae*

    c. Rhinovirus
    d. *Clostridium difficile*
7-3. Which of the following significantly increases the risk of a urinary tract infection?
    a. A history of asthma
    b. An indwelling urinary catheter
    c. Concomitant pneumonia
    d. Recent admission to the hospital
7-4. Which of the following is considered a common nosocomial infection?
    a. Pneumonia
    b. Acute otitis media
    c. Hepatitis
    d. AIDS
7-5. Which of the following factors most significantly contributes to the development of antibiotic resistance?
    a. Indiscriminate antibiotic use
    b. Use of urinary catheters
    c. Mechanical ventilation
    d. Older age

Nosocomial infection is a term used to describe hospital-acquired infection and refers to an infection acquired during one's hospitalization or shortly after discharge from the hospital. The term *health care–associated infection* (HAI) is the definition for any infection that develops as a result of a stay or exposure to a health care facility, including acute or long-term care facilities, free-standing medical centers, dialysis centers, and so forth. HAI is the preferred terminology because patients travel between any or all of these facilities, and it is often impossible to determine the initial source of the infection.

Some microorganisms are pathogenic and have the ability to cause disease or infection in most individuals. But all microorganisms have the potential to cause illness if they access a vulnerable site (blood, surgical wound, etc.) or if the patient's defenses are compromised by invasive procedures, immunosuppressive drugs, or chronic underlying disease.

PATHOPHYSIOLOGY

Many infections are caused by the patient's own skin flora. Often, however, there is a transformation of the normal flora to a more pathogenic flora following admission to a health care facility. Shortly after admission to a health care facility, patients are exposed to various, more virulent strains of the facility's resident flora. This change begins when microorganisms colonize the patient's skin, respiratory, or genitourinary tract. *Colonization* is defined as the presence of a microorganism in a host without causing tissue or cell damage. *Infection* is the presence of microorganism with damage to the host's tissues and/or cells. Colonization always precedes infection but does not necessarily develop into infection.

RISK FACTORS FOR HEALTH CARE–ASSOCIATED INFECTIONS

There are various risk factors for patients in health care facilities. They include invasive procedures such as surgical procedures, vascular and central line placement, urinary catheterization, intubation, and use of antibiotics. Health care workers (HCWs) and patient care staff going from one patient to another may have pathogens on their hands if hand hygiene was not adequate or not done. Many studies have shown that equipment such as stethoscopes can pose a risk for transmission of pathogens.

The environment also plays a critical role in placing patients at risk if cleaning is not adequate. There are studies that implicate contaminated patient environments with the cause of infection. Therefore, housekeeping staff need to be trained to focus on *high touch* areas, or sites that are frequently touched by patients and HCWs, including door knobs, light switches, and call buttons. These sites require thorough cleaning with an FDA-approved detergent or disinfectant. Another environmental risk factor is the close proximity of patients' beds, particularly if patients are immunosuppressed and have an increased length of stay.

High Touch Areas for Environmental Cleaning

- Door knobs
- Light switches
- Bed rails
- Call buttons
- Telephones
- Television remote controls
- Over bed tables
- Toilet handles
- Sink fixtures

PREVENTION

Preventing the transmission of infections is the responsibility of everyone who comes in contact with the patient or the patient's environment. Adverse outcomes of HAI include an increase in patient morbidity and mortality, an increased likelihood of an intensive care unit (ICU) stay, an increased length of stay, increased cost (for which the facility may not receive reimbursement), and an increased probability of readmission.

In order to prevent the spread of infections, it is important to understand and adhere to the U.S. Centers for Disease Control and Prevention (CDC) guidelines regarding standard and transmission-based precautions (CDC, 2007) (see Chapter 1, "Basic Infection Control"). Infection may be spread via direct transmission, which involves touching the patient or the patient's infectious material; or via indirect transmission, which involves touching items contaminated with the patient's infectious material. Ingestion of contaminated food is another route of transmission, but occurrences in a health care setting are uncommon.

While there is much public focus on Methicillin-resistant *Staphylococcus aureus* (MRSA; see Figure 7.1), Vancomycin-resistant enterococci (VRE), and *Clostridium difficile,* resistant gram negatives, are increasingly responsible for HAI. One in particular, *Klebsiella pneumonia,* which is naturally found in soil and is part of the normal human flora of the mouth, skin, and intestines, has developed resistance to many antibiotics. Of particular concern is the Klebsiella strain, which can produce the carbapenemase enzyme, making the organism resistant to the carbapenems. This is critical in that the carbapenems were the last line of treatment for serious gram negative infections. Risks for infection with this organism are mechanical ventilation, as well as central and peripheral intravenous lines. Other multidrug-resistant organisms (MDROs) include the gram negative bacteria of the Acinetobacter and Pseudomonas families. Acinetobacter had long been considered nonpathogenic and an opportunistic pathogen. The organism has the ability for long survival on both wet and dry surfaces, making the health care environment, invasive devices, and medical equipment potential sites for colonization and transmission. *Pseudomonas aeruginosa,* a water-borne organism, is also an opportunistic pathogen, meaning that it exploits some break in the host's defenses to initiate an infection (see Figure 7.2). The bacterium almost never infects uncompromised tissues, yet there is hardly any tissue that it cannot infect if the tissue defenses are compromised in some manner. The organism has the ability to produce biofilm, which increases the risk for bloodstream infections (BSI), central line-associated BSI (CLABSI), and infections related to other invasive devices. It can also cause urinary tract infections (UTIs), catheter-associated UTIs (CAUTIs), respiratory system infections, dermatitis, soft tissue infections, bacteremia, bone and joint infections, gastrointestinal infections, ventilator-associated pneumonia (VAP), and a variety of systemic infections, particularly in patients with severe burns and in those patients who are immunocompromised due to malignancy or AIDS. According to the CDC, the overall incidence of *P. aeruginosa* infections in U.S. hospitals averages about 0.4% (4 per 1,000 discharges), and the bacterium is the fourth most commonly isolated health care–associated pathogen, accounting for 10.1% of all HAIs.

FIGURE 7.1

MRSA wound infection

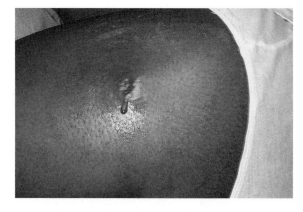

Courtesy of the Centers for Disease Control and Prevention / Bruno Coignard, MD and Jeff Hageman, MHS

FIGURE 7.2

Gram stain of *Pseudomonas aeruginosa*

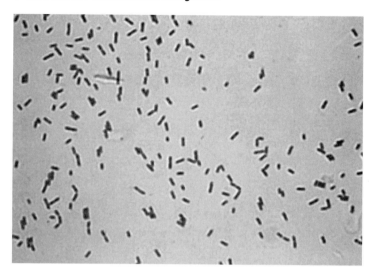

Microorganisms Commonly Seen in HAIs

- *Staphylococcus aureus*
- Methicillin-resistant *Staphylococcus aureus* (MRSA)
- Coagulase-negative Staphylococcus
- Vancomycin-resistant enterococci (VRE)
- *Clostridium difficile*
- Pseudomonas species
- *Klebsiella pneumonia*
- *Acinetobacter baumannii*
- *Serratia marcescens*

WORKUP

Laboratory Studies

A detailed physical examination and review of systems will most likely reveal the involved organs or systems. Investigation should focus on these abnormal areas. Studies should center on infections in the bloodstream (BSI), urinary tract (UTI), and lungs (pneumonia), unless another obvious source (e.g., surgical-site infection [SSI]) is identified. Infections in the ICU have serious consequences and must be monitored (see Table 7.1).

TABLE **7.1**

Frequency of Nosocomial Infections by ICU Type

TYPE OF ICU	CAUTI RATE[1]		CLABSI RATE[2]		VAP RATE[3]	
	Mean	Median	Mean	Median	Mean	Median
Coronary	4.5	4.0	3.5	3.2	4.4	4.0
Cardiothoracic	3.0	2.4	2.7	1.8	7.2	6.3
Medical	5.1	4.7	5.0	3.9	4.9	3.7
Pediatric	4.0	3.6	6.6	5.2	2.9	2.3
Surgical	4.4	3.8	4.6	3.4	9.3	8.3
Trauma	6.0	5.7	7.4	5.2	15.2	11.4

1. $$\text{CAUTI RATE} = \frac{\text{Number of CAUTIs}}{\text{Number of urinary catheter days}} \times 1000$$

2. $$\text{CLABSI RATE} = \frac{\text{Number of CLABSIs}}{\text{Number of central line days}} \times 1000$$

3. $$\text{VAP RATE} = \frac{\text{Number of VAPs}}{\text{Number of ventilator days}} \times 1000$$

Adapted from "National Nosocomial Infections Surveillance (NNIS) System Report, Data Summary from October 1986–April 1998, Issued June 1998," by National Nosocomial Infections Surveillance (NNIS) System, 1998. *American Journal of Infection Control,* 26(5), 522–533.

■ BSI
  ● Obtain quantitative blood cultures with samples from the intravenous line and peripheral vein to aid in differential diagnosis of line-associated BSI. Because of the small volume of blood that is vacuum aspirated into quantitative sample tubes, a regular blood culture is recommended, as this sample may grow the pathogen in cases involving low-inoculum bacteremia.
  ● Fungal cultures should be obtained if fungal infection is suspected. The laboratory will incubate cultures longer for fungal detection than for other microorganisms.
  ● In immunocompromised patients, special studies are occasionally requested, such as cultures for atypical mycobacteria, cytomegalovirus, and cytomegalovirus antigenemia detection.

■ UTI
  ● Patients who have indwelling urinary catheters are at increased risk for developing a CAUTI.
  ● Efforts should be made to differentiate colonization, cystitis, and frank pyelonephritis using urinalysis, urine Gram staining, and culturing.

- Early removal of the urinary catheter is always helpful in the treatment of CAUTI.

◼ Pneumonia
  - Radiography, oxygenation, and hemodynamic status determination are required in the evaluation of nosocomial pneumonia.
  - Examination of the sputum, endotracheal aspiration material, and pleural effusion fluid with gram staining and culturing may be useful.
  - Rapid diagnostic testing may be useful in specific cases. Examples include the direct fluorescent antibody test for *Legionella* organisms or for organisms that cause pertussis; immunofluorescence tests for influenza, respiratory syncytial virus (which is transmitted by contact), and *Pneumocystis jiroveci* (formerly known as *Pneumocystis carinii*); and modified acid-fast stains for mycobacteria.

Treatments of HAI depend on the type and source of infection.

◼ BSI
  - Remove indwelling lines if suspected as the cause of BSI.
  - Select antibiotics according to the local epidemiologic patterns of microbial susceptibility.
  - Add antifungals (e.g., fluconazole, caspofungin, voriconazole, amphotericin B) to empiric antibiotics in appropriate cases.
  - Consider antivirals (e.g., ganciclovir, acyclovir) in the treatment of suspected disseminated viral infections.

◼ UTI
  - Remove indwelling catheters as soon as possible.
  - Administer antimicrobial therapy based on the preliminary results of urinalysis and urine Gram staining.

◼ Pneumonia
  - Change nasotracheal tubes to orotracheal tubes, if feasible.
  - Administer antibiotics with guidance from the results of rapid examination of the sputum, endotracheal suction material, or bronchial lavage wash.
  - Use macrolide antibiotics if legionella is suspected.
  - Consider antiviral medications if viral pneumonia is suspected, especially in symptomatic patients and those who are immunocompromised or have chronic lung diseases to limit morbidity and mortality.
  - Vaccinate against seasonal influenza A and B.

◼ SSI
  - Manage with a combination of surgical care and aggressive antibiotic therapy guided by the results of Gram staining and culturing.
  - Pay special attention to fasciitis given the association with group A streptococci and high morbidity and mortality rates.
  - Débride when necessary.

PREVENTING AND CONTROLLING HAI

It is estimated that approximately one-third of HAI are preventable. Therefore, infection control and prevention are cost-effective. There are three considerations that reduce HAIs:

- Human behavior
- Systems reviews
- Technology

Human Behavior

Among the steps taken to reduce or eliminate transmission of microorganisms, none is more effective than hand washing (see chapter 1, "Basic Infection Control"). The goal of hand washing is to remove microorganisms that might be transmitted to patients, visitors, or other health care personnel. For health care personnel, the CDC recommend that hand washing be done at these times:

- Before performing invasive procedures, whether or not sterile gloves are used
- Before and after contact with any type of wound
- Before contact with particularly susceptible patients, such as those who have diseases that depress the patient's resistance to infectious organisms.
- After contact with body substance or mucous membrane
- Between contact with all patients
- After removing gloves

System Reviews

If each step in any process is so complicated that the slightest deviation will result in an adverse outcome, prevention involves two areas for action.

- Revise the process. How can the number of steps be reduced to prevent overlooking any part of the process?
- Constant and consistent reeducation of staff performing the procedures and monitoring their technique.

Technology

There is constant research going on that is investigating materials for invasive devices and medical equipment. There are silver- and antibiotic-coated catheters, impregnated external patches applied to invasive device sights, and materials for invasive devices that will not support the growth of biofilm.

A successful program to reduce health care–associated infections will include all three components. Another measure to be taken in each facility is monitoring of infections. It is imperative to identify the problem in order to develop a plan for improvement. This monitoring is usually conducted by infection prevention staff using definitions provided by the CDC. No infection prevention program can succeed without addressing antibiotic use. The numbers of resistant organisms are increasing at a rapid rate (see chapter 16, "Antibiotic-Resistant Infections"), therefore antibiotic use must be part of any prevention program.

MRSA of the Skin

HAI are now a target of state and federal governments. Several states have enacted legislation requiring acute care facilities to screen patients for MRSA when they are admitted to the facility or to the intensive care unit. Similar proposals are under consideration for long-term care and rehabilitation facilities.

Some successes in controlling HAIs have come from improving the design of invasive devices, such as catheters. This is particularly important given the marked increase in frequency of vascular access–associated BSIs, particularly in ICU patients. Of particular importance is the development of noninvasive monitoring devices and minimally invasive surgical techniques that avoid the high risk associated with bypassing normal host defense barriers (e.g., the skin and mucous membranes).

Aggressive antibiotic control programs may become mandated for facilities that receive federal reimbursements, as happened in the past with infection control programs. Risks for MDROs may also be reduced in the future by controlling colonization through use of immunization or competing flora.

NURSES' ROLES IN PREVENTING AND CONTROLLING HEALTH CARE–ASSOCIATED INFECTIONS

All HCWs play a critical role in preventing and controlling the spread of infection, especially nurses because they provide a significant amount of direct contact care of the patient. It is imperative that good clinical nursing practice, clear understanding of the infection process, and evidence-based measures to prevent and control the transmission of microorganisms that cause infection be instilled during the introduction to nursing care. The practice of standard precautions, body substance isolation, and medical asepsis are practices that help contain infectious organisms.

Psychosocial Effect

Once a patient is identified as having an infection and placed on isolation precautions appropriate for the mode of transmission, everyone entering and exiting the patient room should follow all recommended practices. This often makes the patient feel as if they are being isolated and not just the organism causing the infection. Strict adherence to wearing protective barriers such as gloves, gowns, and mask combined with limited contact between the HCW and patient may have a negative psychological impact on the patient. The patient may feel dirty and experience a sense of loneliness. It is important for the nurse to be knowledgeable and balance the practice of protective isolation with the emotional support needed to maintain the nurse–patient relationship. The nurse can provide the patient with psychological comfort by not isolating the patient beyond what is necessary. Providing the patient with information about their infection and purpose for protective barriers while listening to their concerns may help to maintain their psychological health.

POST-TEST QUESTIONS

7-1. Which of the following terms refers to a hospital-acquired infection?
   a. Nosocomial
   b. Latent
   c. Smoldering
   d. Active

7-2. An organism commonly associated with health care–associated infections is:
   a. *Haemophilus influenza*
   b. *Streptococcus pneumoniae*
   c. Rhinovirus
   d. *Clostridium difficile*

7-3. Which of the following significantly increases the risk of a urinary tract infection?
   a. A history of asthma
   b. An indwelling urinary catheter
   c. Concomitant pneumonia
   d. Recent admission to the hospital

7-4. Which of the following is considered a common nosocomial infection?
   a. Pneumonia
   b. Acute otitis media
   c. Hepatitis
   d. AIDS

7-5. Which of the following factors most significantly contributes to the development of antibiotic resistance?
   a. Indiscriminate antibiotic use
   b. Use of urinary catheters
   c. Mechanical ventilation
   d. Older age

References

Centers for Disease Control and Prevention (CDC). (2007). Guideline for isolation precautions: Preventing transmission of infectious agents in healthcare settings. Jane D. Siegel, Emily Rhinehart, Marguerite Jackson, Linda Chiarello, the Healthcare Infection Control Practices Advisory Committee. Retrieved April 30, 2010, from http://www.cdc.gov/ncidod/dhqp/pdf/isolation2007.pdf

National Nosocomial Infections Surveillance (NNIS) System. (1998). National Nosocomial Infections Surveillance (NNIS) System report, data summary from October 1986–April 1998, issued June 1998. *American Journal of Infection Control, 26* (5), 522–533.

Web Sites

http://phil.cdc.gov/phil/home.asp

Suggested Reading

Bischoff, W.E., et al. (2000). Handwashing compliance by health care workers: The impact of introducing an accessible, alcohol-based hand antiseptic. *Archives of Internal Medicine, 160*.

Bratus, L. D, Haag, R., Recco, R., Eramo, A., Alam, M., & Quale, J. (2005). Rapid spread of carbapenem-resistant Klebsiella pneumonia in New York City: A new threat to our antibiotic armamentarium. *Archives of Internal Medicine, 165*(12), 1430–1435.

Centers for Disease Control and Prevention. (2009). *What you should know about Klebsiella infections.* Retrieved August 9, 2009, from http://www.cdc.gov/ncidod/dhqp/ar_kp_about.html

Dancer, S.J. (1999). Mopping up hospital infection. *Journal of Hospital Infection, 43*(2), 85–100.

Deville, J.G., Adler, S., Azimi, P.H., Jantausch, B. A., Morfin, M. R., Beltran, S., et al. (2003). Linezolid versus vancomycin in the treatment of known or suspected resistant gram-positive infections in neonates. *Pediatric Infectious Disease Journal, 22*(9 Suppl), S158–S163.

Donlan, R.M. (2001). Biofilms and device-associated infections. *CDC Emerging Infectious Diseases, 7*(2), 277–281.

Garner, J.S. (1996). Guideline for isolation precautions in hospitals. The Hospital Infection Control Practices Advisory Committee [published erratum appears in 1996, *Infection Control and Hospital Epidemiology, 17*(4), 214]. *Infection Control and Hospital Epidemiology, 17*(1), 53–80.

McKibben, L., Horan, T., Tokars, J., Fowler, G., Cardo, D., Pearson, M., et al. (2005). Guidance on public reporting of healthcare-associated infections: Recommendations of the Healthcare Infection Control Practices Advisory Committee. *Am J Infect Control, 33*(4), 217–226.

Merlin, M. A., Wong, M. L., Pryor, P. W., Rynn, K., Marques-Baptista, A., Perritt, R., et al. (2009). Prevalence of Methicillin-resistant *Staphylococcus aureus* on the stethoscopes of emergency medical services providers. *Prehospital Emergency Care, 13*(1), 71–74.

Richards, M.J., Edwards, J.R., Culver, D.H., & Gaynes, R.P. (1999). Nosocomial infections in pediatric intensive care units in the United States. National Nosocomial Infections Surveillance System. *Pediatrics, 103*(4), e39.

Tenover, F.C., Kalsi, R. K., Williams, P. P., Carey, R. B., Stocker, S., Lonsway, D., et al. (2006). Carbapenem resistance in *Klebsiella pneumonia* not detected by automated susceptibility testing. *Emerging Infectious Diseases, 12*(8), 1209–1213.

Wenzel, R., & Edmond, M.D. (2001). The impact of hospital acquired blood stream infections. *Emerging Infectious Diseases, 7*(2), 174–177.

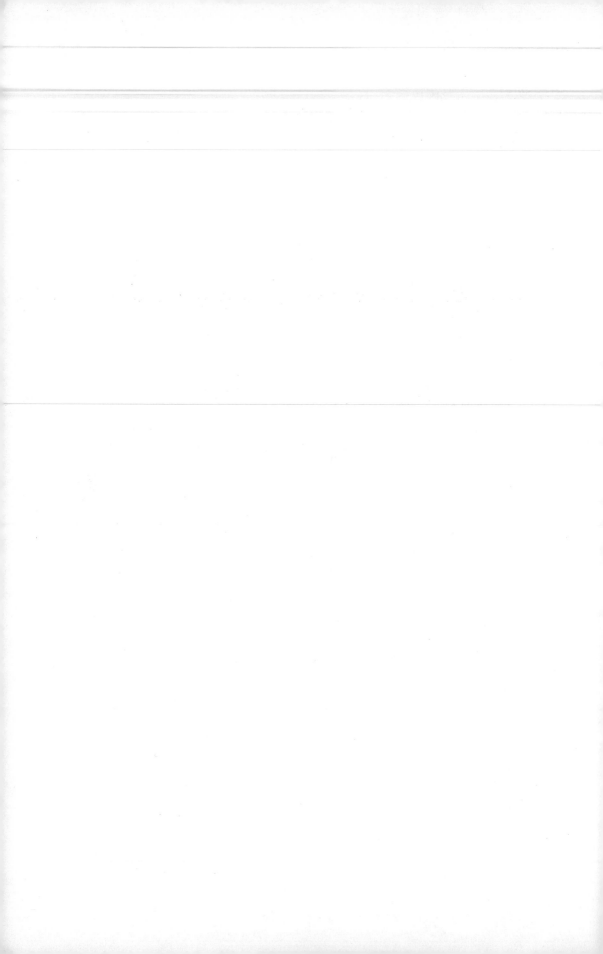

8

Infection Control in Critical Care

This chapter includes topics on the epidemiology of infection in the burn unit and critical care unit. The ventilator-associated pneumonias are reviewed. The content discusses the different stages of decubitus ulcers. The staging criteria for decubitus ulcers as well as clinical indications of methods to control urinary catheter infections are reviewed. Finally, device-related blood stream infections and soft tissue infections are discussed.

OBJECTIVES

1. Identify the epidemiology of infection in the burn unit.
2. Describe strategies for infection prevention and control.
3. List three common infections seen in patients in the critical care unit.
4. List three methods to reduce ventilator-associated pneumonia.
5. Understand the staging criteria for a decubitus ulcer.

PRE-TEST QUESTIONS

8-1. The most important risk factor for the development of a catheter-associated urinary tract infection is:
   a. Duration of urinary catheter placement
   b. Age of the patient
   c. Underlying illnesses
   d. Primary diagnosis

8-2. Which of the following statements is true regarding antimicrobial prophylaxis and surgical site infections?
   a. Antibiotics should be administered at least 2 hours prior to the incision.

    b. For procedures lasting more than 2 hours, a second dose of the antibiotic may be warranted.

    c. For surgical procedures involving implants, antibiotic prophylaxis is unnecessary.

    d. The type of surgical procedure affects the antibiotic used for antimicrobial prophylaxis.

8-3. Risk factors for infection in a patient with significant burns include:

    a. Increase of virulent pathogens in the burn unit

    b. Altered barrier of immunity

    c. Use of many immunosuppressive medications

    d. Malnutrition

8-4. Which of the following is a method to reduce the incidence of ventilator-associated pneumonia?

    a. Increase the duration of time the patient is receiving mechanical ventilation.

    b. Use an endotracheal tube with a dorsal lumen.

    c. Use a naso-tracheal tube instead of an oro-tracheal tube in patients that require mechanical ventilation.

    d. Use endotracheal intubation instead of noninvasive ventilation.

8-5. Visitors to the burn unit:

    a. Should wash their hands before entering the burn unit

    b. May bring flowers to the patient

    c. May be allowed even if they have signs of infections

    d. May bring fresh fruit to the patient to speed their healing

Patients that are admitted to critical care units are among the sickest and most vulnerable hospitalized patients (see Figure 8.1). These individuals are at the highest risk for complications if they acquire health care–associated infections (HAIs). They usually have concurrent organ system dysfunction, such as heart, liver, or kidney failure, and may also suffer from an altered immune response. Additionally, these patients are treated with multiple medical devices, such as mechanical ventilators, diagnostic catheters (for arterial, venous, and intracranial pressure monitoring), therapeutic catheters (both central and peripherally inserted) used for medications and other therapies, such as dialysis, drainage catheters (rectal and bladder), and enteral feeding tubes, as well as hemodynamic stabilization devices, such as intraaortic balloon pump, left ventricular assist devices, pacemakers, and defibrillators (see Figure 8.2).

These patients are cohorted into a common area, the critical, or intensive, care unit, in order to separate them from other hospitalized patients who are less severely ill. While this may help to consolidate resources, it also creates the perfect environment for the transmission of infection, including those caused by multidrug resistant organisms (MDROs). As in all areas of health care, adherence to the basic tenets of hand washing (see Chapter 1, "Basic Infection Control") is crucial. Health care workers (HCWs), such as nurses, intensivists, respiratory therapists, physical and occupational therapists, pharmacists, and even housekeeping staff, move from room to room, coming into contact with potentially infected patients and surfaces (see Figure 8.3). Surface decontamination and correct use of personal protective equipment (PPE) are necessary to keep patients and staff

FIGURE 8.1

Critical care patient

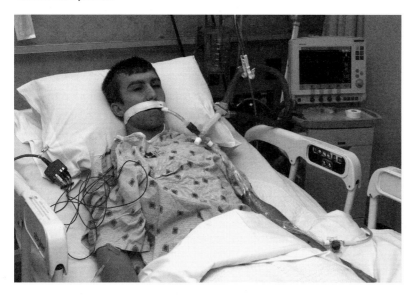

FIGURE 8.2

Critical care patient with multiple medical devices, such as mechanical ventilation, diagnostic catheters (for arterial, venous, and intracranial pressure monitoring), therapeutic catheters (both central and peripherally inserted) used for medications

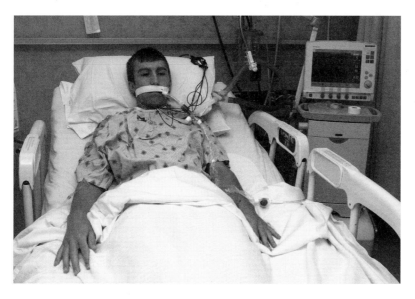

FIGURE 8.3

Respiratory therapists come into contact with potentially infected patients

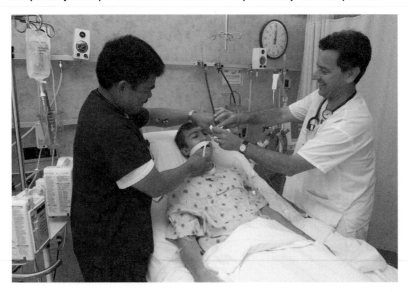

healthy. In addition, visitors must also be educated on hand washing and use of alcohol-based gels upon entering and exiting the unit. Signs and brochures (see Appendix) are an excellent means to teach family members and visitors to use proper infection control practices.

Infections in the critical care unit include catheter-associated urinary tract infections (CAUTI), ventilator-associated pneumonias (VAPs), device-related blood stream infections (BSIs), and skin and soft tissue infections, such as decubitus ulcers and surgical site infections (SSIs). According to the Centers for Disease Control and Prevention (CDC), HAIs are one of the top 10 leading causes of death in the United States. The CDC estimates that there are 1.7 million HAIs in American hospitals each year, with 99,000 associated deaths (Department of Health and Human Services [DHHS], Centers for Medicare and Medicaid Services [CMS], 2007)

HCWs and hospitals can reduce patient risk by adopting and implementing standards of evidence-based best practices. This is both sound patient care and financial advice. In 2009, Medicare announced that it will no longer cover the costs of "preventable" conditions, mistakes, and infections resulting from a hospital stay. So if you are in the hospital and on Medicare and you develop a HAI, such as a *Staphlococcal aureus* wound infection (see Figure 8.4), while being treated post-operatively for a surgery to remove a growth, Medicare will not pay that portion of the bill. According to a statement from the Centers for Medicare and Medicaid Services (CMS), the new rule is part of a step to: "Improve the accuracy of Medicare's payment under the acute care hospital inpatient prospective payment system (IPPS), while providing additional incentives for hospitals to engage in quality improvement efforts" (Medical News Today, 2007).

FIGURE 8.4

Staphlococcal aureus wound infection

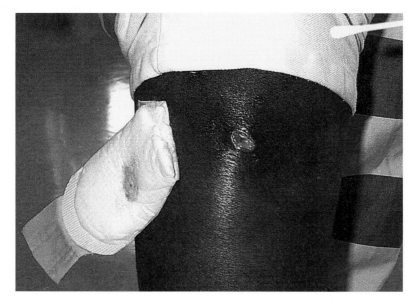

Courtesy of the Centers for Disease Control and Prevention / Bruno Coignard, MD and Jeff Hageman, MHS

CATHETER-ASSOCIATED URINARY TRACT INFECTION (CAUTI)

CAUTI is the most common infection acquired by hospitalized adult patients, accounting for 30%–40% of all HAIs. In the hospital, the critical care unit has the highest prevalence of CAUTI, representing up to 21% of HAIs. While a urinary tract infection is usually considered a mild illness, it can become more severe and result in pyelonephritis or produce urosepsis. These infections can increase the cost of care, length of stay, and mortality rate.

Most commonly, hospital-acquired UTIs are caused by *E. coli* and other aerobic gram negative enteric organisms. These organisms are becoming increasingly more resistant to antibiotics and pose a therapeutic challenge. A number of techniques have been suggested to reduce the incidence of CAUTIs in patients who are critically ill. For example, catheters should only be used when clinically indicated, placed using the aseptic technique, and used for the shortest time necessary with closed drainage system. The duration of catheterization is the most important risk factor in the development of CAUTIs.

Clinical Indications for Urinary Catheters

- Perioperative for selected procedures
- Measuring urine output in critically ill patients
- Management of acute urinary retention/urinary obstruction

- Assistance in pressure ulcer healing for incontinent patients
- Comfort in end-of-life care

Silver-coated catheters may reduce the rate of nosocomial urinary tract infections. However, these catheters are more expensive than non–silver-coated catheters. Methods that have not been shown to reduce catheter-associated infections include bladder irrigation, antibacterial agents in collection bag, and rigorous meatal cleaning. Other urine collection strategies, such as intermittent catheterization, suprapubic catheterization, and the use of a condom catheter, have also been suggested as a method to reduce the incidence of CAUTIs.

VENTILATOR-ASSOCIATED PNEUMONIA (VAP)

Pneumonia accounts for approximately 25% of all infections reported in the critical care unit and is the second most common HAI. Hospital-acquired pneumonia occurs at a rate of 5–10 cases per 1,000 admissions and prolongs hospital length of stay (LOS) by more than 1 week. The overwhelming majority of episodes of pneumonia seen in critical care are associated with mechanical ventilation, resulting in ventilator-associated pneumonia (VAP) (American Thoracic Society, Infectious Diseases Society of America, 2005) (see Figure 8.5).

Early-onset VAP typically occurs within 4 days after intubation and is most commonly caused by *Streptococcus pneumoniae, Haemophilus influenzae,* and an-

FIGURE 8.5

The overwhelming majority of episodes of pneumonia seen in critical care are associated with mechanical ventilation, resulting in ventilator-associated pneumonia

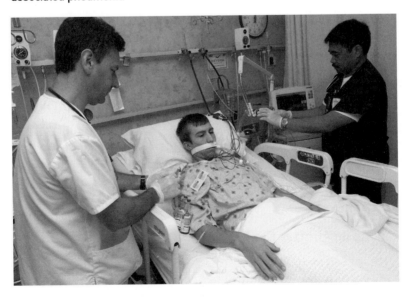

aerobic microorganisms. Conversely, late-onset VAP occurs more than 4 days after intubation and is more commonly associated with hospital-associated pathogens, such as *Pseudomonas aeruginosa, Acinetobacter spp, Enterobacter spp, Staphylo-coccus aureus,* and enteric microorganisms. Fungal infections involving *Candida spp.* and *Aspergillus spp.* occur in less than 10% of cases.

Risk factors for the development of VAP include endotracheal suctioning, aerosol treatments, collection of subglottal secretions, presence of nasogastric tube, stress ulcer prophylaxis using antacids / H2 blockers / proton pump inhibitors (PPIs), and corticosteroid therapy. In May 2004, the CDC released guidelines for the prevention of healthcare–associated pneumonias.

Methods to Reduce VAP

- Reduction of the duration of mechanical ventilation
- Preferential use of oro-tracheal rather than naso-tracheal tubes in patients who receive mechanically assisted ventilation
- Use of noninvasive ventilation to reduce the need for and duration of endotracheal intubation
- Changing the breathing circuits of ventilators when they malfunction or are visibly contaminated
- When feasible, the use of an endotracheal tube with a dorsal lumen to allow drainage of respiratory secretions

DEVICE-RELATED BLOOD STREAM INFECTION (BSI)

Almost all hospitalized patients have an intravascular device at some point during their hospital admission. Roughly half of all patients admitted to the critical care unit have a central vein catheter (CVC). CVCs result in 80,000 infections per year, which increase patient mortality, hospital LOS, and cost. The CDC defines a catheter-related BSI as one that occurs in a patient with a vascular access device that was in place in the 48-hour period before the BSI developed, and the device was indwelling for more than a 48-hour duration, with no other source of infection. Catheter cultures may be obtained using either the roll plate method or the broth culture method after the catheter tip has been retrieved. In the roll plate method, the catheter tip is rolled onto a culture-media plate. Colony counts greater than 15 colony forming units (cfu) are considered positive. The broth culture method involves either flushing the catheter tip or immersing the tip in a culture broth media. More than 103 cfu is considered to be a positive result. The roll plate method typically only identifies microorganisms growing on the outside of the catheter. The broth method only identifies microorganisms growing on the inside of the catheter, if the catheter tip is flushed into the broth media. If the tip is flushed and immersed with broth culture medium, microorganisms growing on the inside and outside can be identified.

Method for Retrieving Catheter Tip for Culture

- Don sterile gown, gloves, and mask.
- Prep catheter site with antiseptic agent according to unit protocol.

- Remove catheter sutures using sterile scissors.
- Withdraw catheter while holding pressure using sterile gauze.
- Insert catheter tip into sterile specimen cup (do not let catheter come in contact with any nonsterile item).
- Cut an approximate 2-inch segment using sterile scissors.

There are several different types of CVCs (see Figures 8.6–8.18). These account for the majority of catheter-related BSIs. Pulmonary artery catheters enter the vascular system via an introducer (that is not tunneled) and have infection rates similar to nontunneled CVCs. Peripherally inserted central catheters (PICCs) are nontunneled catheters that enter the vascular system via a peripheral vein (usually the brachial or basilic vein) with the catheter tip ending in a central vessel. These devices have lower rates of BSI compared with nontunneled CVCs. Tunneled CVCs penetrate the skin at a site that is distant from the vascular entry site. The catheter extends in a subcutaneous "tunnel" between the catheter exit site and the vascular entry site. Tunneled catheters (sometimes referred to as cuffed-catheters) have a synthetic cuff that forms a biomechanic barrier when endothelial cells grow into the cuff material. The cuff is positioned between the catheter exit site and the tunnel, thereby reducing the possibility that skin microorganisms can gain entry into the blood stream via the catheter. Tunneled catheters have a lower BSI rate compared with nontunneled catheters. Totally implantable catheters have no external components. These are both placed and removed surgically and have the lowest rates of catheter-related BSI.

Device-related BSIs can be prevented. Review indications for device placement. All devices must be inserted using strict sterile technique as would be

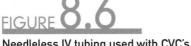

FIGURE 8.6

Needleless IV tubing used with CVC's

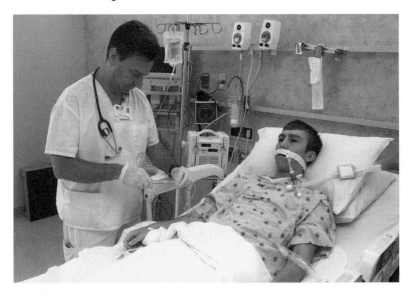

FIGURE 8.7

Needleless IV tubing to prevent healthcare worker needlestick injuries

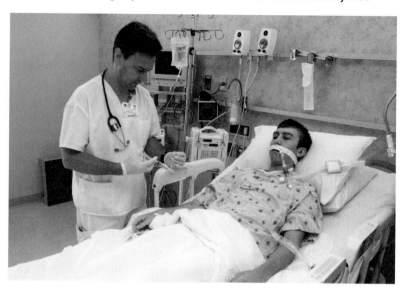

FIGURE 8.8

Drawing blood cultures from a triple lumen central venous catheter

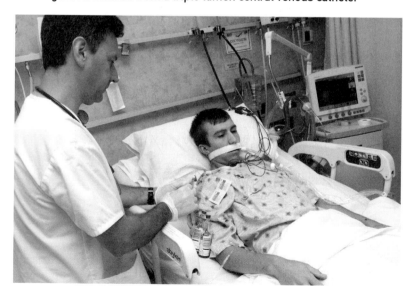

FIGURE 8.9

Tubing labels (yellow)
change date is for IV tubing

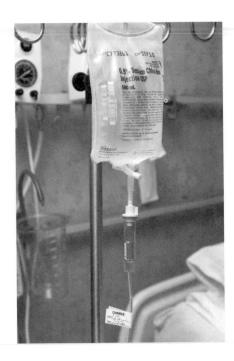

FIGURE 8.10

Implanted port reservoir

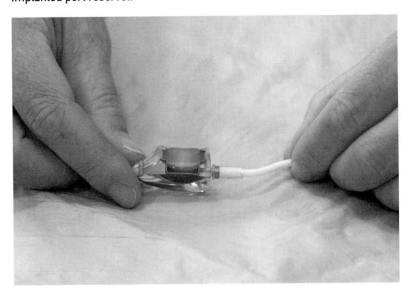

FIGURE 8.11
Dual-lumen implanted port

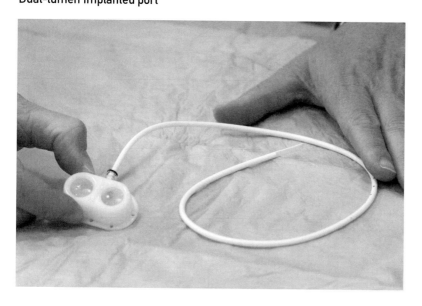

FIGURE 8.12
Triple-lumen short term central venous catheter (CVC)

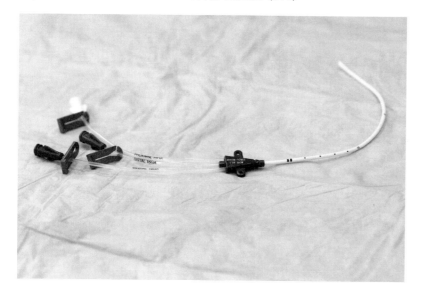

FIGURE **8.13**

Power injection peripherally inserted central catheter (PICC)

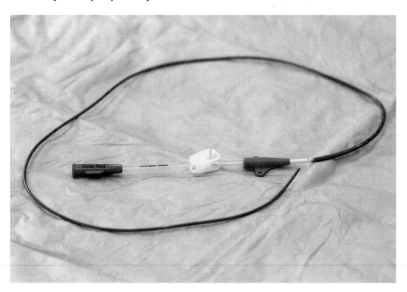

FIGURE **8.14**

Dialysis catheter

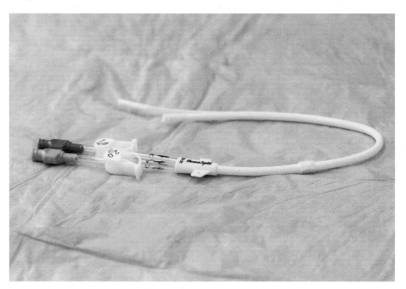

FIGURE 8.15

Single-lumen power implanted subcutaneous power port

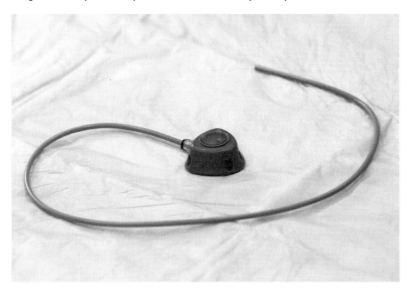

FIGURE 8.16

Non-coring implanted port needle

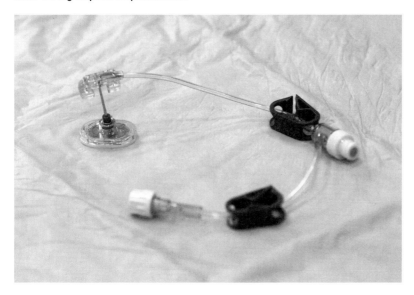

FIGURE **8.17**

Dual-lumen Groshing PICC

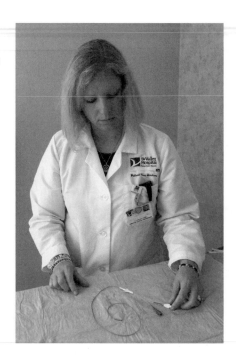

FIGURE **8.18**

Triple-lumen power injected PICC

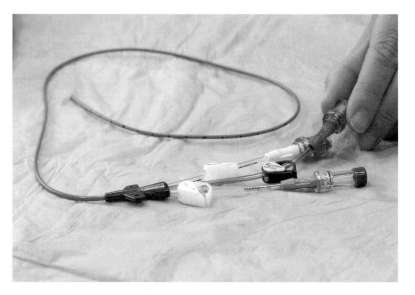

performed in the operating room. Hands must be sanitized. Maximum barrier precautions must be observed using gloves, gown, cap, and mask for everyone in the room; skin antisepsis using chlorhexidine gluconate rather than iodophors; and prompt removal of device when indication for placement has resolved. Examine all device sites by inspection and palpation for the signs and symptoms of infection, including tenderness, erythema, warmth, and discharge. Monitor the patient for fever, chills, hemodynamic alterations, and confusion.

SOFT TISSUE INFECTIONS

Decubitus ulcers often occur in patients who are critically ill. These lesions occur because of prolonged pressure that cuts off the blood supply to the skin, causing the skin and other tissue to die. The damage may occur in as little time as 1 to 2 hours of pressure. This most commonly occurs in patients who cannot move by themselves, such as patients who are paralyzed or have suffered from a stroke.

There are a number of risk factors for the development of decubitus ulcers. The skin is especially likely to develop pressure sores if it is exposed to friction shear forces, as in sliding down when the bed head is raised. This is especially true in the elderly because the skin is thinner and is more prone to tearing with simple shear force. Dampness (such as from perspiration or incontinence) makes the skin even more liable to develop pressure sores. Attention to and prevention of these risk factors is vital.

Initially, the area where a decubitus ulcer is forming becomes red. This then progresses to a breakdown in the integrity of the skin, leading to an open wound, which may be oozing. The areas most prone to decubitus formation are areas where there is increased pressure, such as the tailbone (coccyx) or buttocks area, shoulder blades, spine, heels, or backs of the arms or legs.

Bedsores are categorized in stages (see Figure 8.19).

In decubitus ulcers that are in stage 1 or 2, treatment involves relief of pressure and care to the affected skin. To relieve pressure patients should be rotated frequently (every 15 minutes in a chair and every 2 hours in a bed). In addition, the use of soft materials or supports (pads, cushions, and mattresses) may reduce pressure against the skin. If the skin is not broken, the area should be gently washed with mild soap and water. The area can also be protected by a thin layer of petroleum jelly and a soft gauze dressing. It is important to keep the area dry and clean. Prolonged contact of the area with urine and stool should be avoided.

In more severe cases of decubitus ulcers (stages 3 and 4), special dressings may be used, and whirlpool baths or surgery may be recommended to remove dead tissue. Infection, if present, requires antibiotic treatment. Sometimes deep wounds may require surgery to restore the tissue. Experimental work is now being done using honey preparations, hyperbaricoxygen, and application of growth factors.

Complications of decubitus ulcers include cellulitis, bone and joint infections, and sepsis. Cellulitis is an acute infection of the skin. Cellulitis can also lead to life-threatening complications, including bone and joint infections and sepsis. If an infection is present, either oral or intravenous antibiotics are necessary.

FIGURE **8.19**

Decubitus ulcers

Stage 1—Skin is unbroken, but pink or ashen (in darker skin) discoloration. May have slight itch or tenderness

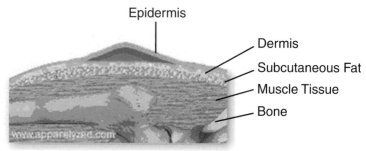

Epidermis
Dermis
Subcutaneous Fat
Muscle Tissue
Bone

Stage 2—Skin has red, swollen areas with a blister or open areas

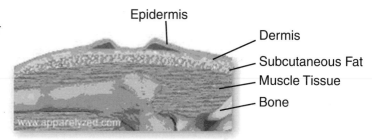

Epidermis
Dermis
Subcutaneous Fat
Muscle Tissue
Bone

Stage 3—Skin has crater-like ulcer extending deeper into the skin

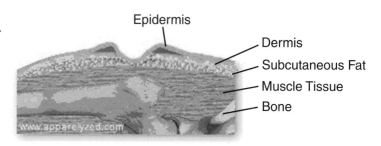

Epidermis
Dermis
Subcutaneous Fat
Muscle Tissue
Bone

Stage 4—Ulcer extends to deep fat, muscle, or bone and may have a thick black scab (eschar)

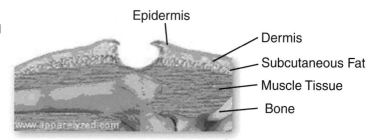

Epidermis
Dermis
Subcutaneous Fat
Muscle Tissue
Bone

SURGICAL SITE INFECTIONS (SSI)

Patients in the critical care unit often have at least one surgical procedure, which may result in infection. SSIs are the third most commonly reported HAI. These infections are the cause of significant morbidity for critical care patients and increase the use of antibiotics, as well as the LOS and mortality rate.

SSIs most commonly occur within 30 days of the surgical procedure and can involve the skin, subcutaneous or deep soft tissue. Patients may complain of pain, tenderness, localized swelling, redness or warmth of the site, or fever. A purulent discharge may be visible.

Prevention of surgical site infections involve the operating room environment and attire, proper cleaning of surgical equipment, hair removal, antiseptic skin preparation, antimicrobial prophylaxis, and post-operative care.

The environment of the operating room must be carefully controlled. For example, the temperature should be between 68 degrees and 73 degrees F, and the humidity should be maintained between 30% and 60%. The operating room should be a positive pressure environment, and air should be introduced from the ceiling and exhausted at the floor. Operating room attire should consist of masks to cover the nose and mouth, caps or hoods to cover head and facial hair, scrub suits, and shoe covers. Drapes used during the surgical procedure must be impermeable to liquids and microorganisms. All equipment must be sterile.

Preparation of the surgical site is another important step in infection control. If hair removal is deemed necessary, only hair that is directly over the surgical site should be removed. This should be done using clippers, not razors, and hair removal should be performed immediately prior to the surgical procedure (not the night before). Antisepsis of the skin can be achieved through the use of iodophors such as povidone-iodine, alcohol-containing products, or chlorhexidine.

Up to one-half of all surgical site infections are preventable with the appropriate use of prophylactic antibiotics. However, overuse, underuse, improper timing, and misuse of antibiotics are rampant and can lead to unnecessary infections. When selecting the antibiotic for prophylaxis, the likely contaminating organisms should be considered. For example, in a surgical procedure involving the bowels, an antibiotic effective against gram negative and anaerobic microorganisms should be used. Antibiotics should be administered between 30 minutes to 2 hours prior to the incision. For procedures lasting more than 4 hours, a second dose of the antibiotic may be warranted. For surgical procedures involving implants, a longer duration of antimicrobial therapy is needed, and patients should receive three doses of the antibiotic over the 18-hour post-operative period.

INFECTION CONTROL IN BURN UNIT

While infection control in the burn unit shares many general principles with other intensive care units, there are a number of issues that are unique to the burn unit. The burn unit is a unique situation in that the patients are at an increased susceptibility because of the altered barrier of immunity, the skin, and altered physiological states. The importance of infection control cannot be stressed enough because it is the leading cause of morbidity and mortality in the burn unit.

The body's natural defenses against infection are (1) physical defenses and (2) immune responses, which could be specific and nonspecific. Changes in these defenses determine the burn patient's *susceptibility* to infection. For example, patient factors such as age (greater than 60 and less than 2 years old), burn area (greater than 30% of total body surface area), full thickness burn, and comorbidities (e.g., diabetes, renal failure) are important considerations that increase the patient's susceptibility to infection (see Figure 8.20). In addition, physiological changes such as dehydration, metabolic and electrolyte disturbances, and high levels of circulating corticosteroids all contribute to diminished resistance to infection.

In the burn patient, the *mode of transmission* is primarily via direct contact with the caregivers' hands and improperly disinfected equipment, for example, hydrotherapy tanks. Indirectly, transmission could be via droplet and airborne spread. Organisms that have been associated with the burn patient include gram-positive organisms that initially colonize the wound, gram-negative organisms, and fungi. Of particular importance are the gram-positive organisms that include methicillin-resistant *Staphylococcus aureus* (MRSA) and vancomycin-resistant enterococcus (VRE), which have become increasingly endemic in burn units.

The goals of infection control and prevention in the burn unit should be based on the knowledge of the sources and modes of transmission of organisms, as described previously. Therefore, the goals should include (1) control of transfer

FIGURE 8.20

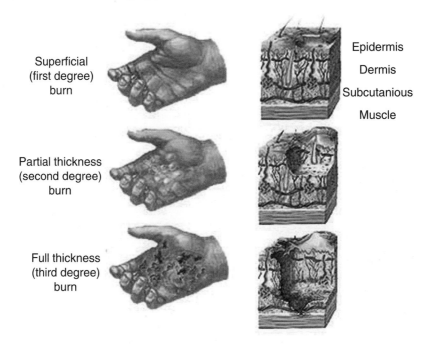

Superficial (first degree) burn

Partial thickness (second degree) burn

Full thickness (third degree) burn

Epidermis

Dermis

Subcutanious

Muscle

of endogenous organisms to the burn sites and (2) prevention of transfer of exogenous organisms from other persons (caregivers, visitors, and other patients) and equipment.

Basic infection control principles, including hand hygiene, and appropriate use of PPE for both HCW and visitors are vital in a burn unit (see Chapter 1, "Basic Infection Control" and Figure 8.21). In addition, the facility or the burn unit should be physically separated from other areas where single rooms are provided for isolation. The unit should have no direct airflow with other areas/wards. Air should be filtered at positive pressure into individual rooms and extracted to the exterior. Isolation precautions in addition to standard precautions should be observed in patients with more than 30% total body surface area burned and those with MDROs.

Wound care, including dressing, should be performed observing aseptic technique, preferably done on bedside. Barrier technique (gown, glove, and mask) should be observed. Expose, clean, and rewrap less infected areas first. Wound swabs for culture must be taken from different burn areas on admission or transfer in and as ordered. Culture and sensitivity reports should be monitored and referred to accordingly.

Environmental hygiene should include daily mopping of furniture, bedside lamps, and door handles or knobs. No sharing of washbowls or furniture, for example, beds and chairs. Whirlpool is not recommended for routine use, however, the whirlpool and shower must be disinfected between patient uses. Items that cannot be effectively decontaminated, such as stuffed toys, should be restricted. Live plants and flowers are not permitted in the burn unit. Linen agitation should

FIGURE 8.21

Basic infection control principles, including hand hygiene, and appropriate use of PPE for both HCW and visitors are vital in a burn unit

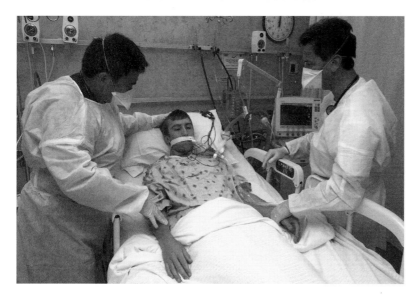

be minimized, and soiled linen should be placed in hampers promptly. All equipment, materials, and surfaces used for or on a patient are considered contaminated and should be decontaminated and stored properly before circulation (see Chapter 6, "Safe Patient Handling and Movement").

All visitors should be oriented to the burn unit's infection control practices (i.e., hand washing, gowning, and isolation precautions), and compliance of such should be monitored. Visitors should be screened for infection, and those found to be potentially infected should be restricted. Also, the number of visitors present at one time should be limited.

Hand washing should be done before and after each patient contact with soap and water, or an antiseptic hand rub could be an alternative for hands without visible dirt. Hand washing also should be done after removing gloves.

Gloving (see Chapter 1, "Basic Infection Control" for a detailed discussion about gloving) should be observed when in contact with blood, body fluids, secretions, and excretions. Gloves should be changed when contaminated with secretions or excretions from one site prior to contact with another site, even if care of the patient is not completed. Sterile gloves should be worn for wound dressing.

A protective gown or apron should be worn to prevent soiling and inapparent contamination of personal uniform, which could then be transmitted to other patients or personnel.

Nutritional support should be enforced to each burn patient. Oral and enteral feeding should be encouraged, and avoid parenteral alimentation (risk of cannula-associated infection). If no diet contraindications exist, a high-protein, high-calorie diet should be encouraged.

POST-TEST QUESTIONS

8-1. The most important risk factor for the development of a catheter-associated urinary tract infection is:
   a. Duration of urinary catheter placement
   b. Age of the patient
   c. Underlying illnesses
   d. Primary diagnosis

8-2. Which of the following statements is true regarding antimicrobial prophylaxis and surgical site infections?
   a. Antibiotics should be administered at least 2 hours prior to the incision.
   b. For procedures lasting more than 2 hours, a second dose of the antibiotic may be warranted.
   c. For surgical procedures involving implants, antibiotic prophylaxis is unnecessary.
   d. The type of surgical procedure affects the antibiotic used for antimicrobial prophylaxis.

8-3. Risk factors for infection in a patient with significant burns include:
   a. Increase of virulent pathogens in the burn unit
   b. Altered barrier of immunity

    c. Use of many immunosuppressive medications

    d. Malnutrition

8-4. Which of the following is a method to reduce the incidence of ventilator associated pneumonia?

    a. Increase the duration of time the patient is receiving mechanical ventilation.

    b. Use an endotracheal tube with a dorsal lumen.

    c. Use a naso-tracheal tube instead of an oro-tracheal tube in patients that require mechanical ventilation.

    d. Use endotracheal intubation instead of noninvasive ventilation.

8-5. Visitors to the burn unit:

    a. Should wash their hands before entering the burn unit

    b. May bring flowers to the patient

    c. May be allowed even if they have signs of infections

    d. May bring fresh fruit to the patient to speed their healing

References

American Thoracic Society, Infectious Diseases Society of America. (2005). Guidelines for the management of adults with hospital-acquired, ventilator-associated, and healthcare-associated pneumonia. American Journal of Respiratory & Critical Care Medicine. 171(4): 388-416.

Centers for Disease Control and Prevention. (2004). Guidelines for preventing health-care–associated pneumonia, 2003. MMWR, 53(RR03), 1–36. Retrieved from http://www.cdc.gov/mmwr/preview/mmwrhtml/rr5303a1.htm

Department of Health & Human Services, Centers for Medicare & Medicaid Services. (2007). Revisions to the hospital interpretive guidelines for infection control. Retrieved October 6, 2009, from http://www.cms.hhs.gov/SurveyCertificationGenInfo/downloads/SCLetter08-04.pdf

Medical News Today. (2007). Medicare will not pay for hospital mistakes and infections, new rule. Retrieved October 6, 2009, from http://www.medicalnewstoday.com/articles/80074.php

Additional Resources

Church, D., Elsayed, S., Reid, O., Winston, B., and Lindsay, R. Burn Wound Infections. Clinical Microbiology Reviews, Volume 19, No. 2, April 2006, Pages 403–434.

Gibran NS, Committee on Organization and Delivery of Burn Care, American Burn Association. Practice guidelines for burn care, 2006. J Burn Care Res. 2006; 27: 437–438.

Husain, M.T. Karim, Q.N., and Tajuri, S., Analysis of infection in a burn ward. Burns, Volume 15, Issue 5, October 1989, Pages 299–302.

Working party report. Principles of design of burn units: report of a Working Group of the British Burn Association and Hospital Infection Society. Journal of Hospital Infection, Volume 19, Issue 1, September 1991, Pages 63–66.

Web Sites

http://www.apparelyzed.com/pressuresores.html

http://www.burn-recovery.org/images/burn-classification.jpg

Infection Control in Labor and Delivery

9

This chapter includes topics on perinatal infections and the prevention and treatment of puerperal infections. The TORCH infections affecting newborns are reviewed. The content discusses ways to prevent newborn infections. There is discussion on the causes of fever in the puerperal period, toxoplasmosis, chlamydia, gonorrhea, rubella, cytomegalovirus (CMV), omphaliitis, and syphilis.

OBJECTIVES

1. Discuss general perinatal infection control issues.
2. Discuss the prevention and treatment of puerperal infection.
3. List TORCH infections affecting newborns.
4. Identify preventative care measures for the infant.
5. Define group B Streptococcal disease (GBS).

PRE-TEST QUESTIONS

9-1. One of the main post-operative infections seen after caesarean section surgery is:
   a. Endometritis
   b. Episiotomy infection
   c. Hepatitis B infection
   d. Chlamydia infection

9-2. Which of the following describes a breast infection?
   a. Toxoplasmosis
   b. Thrombophlebitis
   c. Atelectasis
   d. Mastitis

9-3. Which of the following organisms can cause eye infections in the neonate if routine eye infection prophylaxis is not administered?

a. Group B streptococcus

b. *Neiserria gonorrhea*

c. Herpes simplex virus

d. Cytomegalovirus

9-4. TORCH is an acronym for:

a. Tularemia, other infections, rickettsia, cytomegalovirus, herpes simplex virus

b. Tularemia, other infections, rubella, chlamydia, herpes simplex virus

c. Toxoplasmosis, other infections, rubella, cytomegalovirus, herpes simplex virus

d. Toxoplasmosis, other infections, rubella, cytomegalovirus, herpes zoster virus

9-5. All of the following are vaccine-preventable illnesses that can spread to the neonate during pregnancy or during delivery *except*:

a. Chlamydia

b. Rubella

c. Varicella

d. Hepatitis B

Infection control is imperative in the perinatal unit. Many infections for the mother and baby are health care–associated infections (HAI), with pathogen acquired from the hospital environment. A neonatal HAI is considered an infection that develops within 48 hours of delivery (Gilstrap & Oh, 2002). Many infections in mother and baby are acquired from organisms that are indigenous to the female genital tract, but are "neither present nor incubating when the patient is admitted to the hospital," and are therefore considered HAIs (Gilstrap & Oh, 2002, p. 331).

The approach to preventing perinatal infections must cross all hospital disciplines, with strict adherence to infection control and prevention policies. Meticulous patient care techniques, along with the proper use of antibiotics, will greatly reduce infection rates (Gilstrap & Oh, 2002).

Hand washing is the most important element in the control of infection (see Chapter 1, "Basic Infection Control"). "Handwashing before and after each patient contact remains the single most important routine practice in the control of nosocomial infections" (Gilstrap & Oh, 2002, p. 336). Upon entering the nursery in the beginning of a shift, health care workers (HCWs) need to scrub their hands and arms, above the elbow, for a total of 3 minutes using an antiseptic soap (Gilstrap & Oh, 2002). Disposable brushes and pads, foot pedals controlling water flow, and drying hands with paper towels are helpful in preventing contamination. After the initial scrub, HCWs need to do a 10-second brushless wash with bactericidal soap, before and after handling any neonate. Chlorhexidine gluconate (4%) and iodophor preparation are the bactericidal agents routinely used for hand washing (Gilstrap & Oh, 2002). HCWs need to remove all hand and wrist jewelry, keep fingernails short, and use clear nail polish with only natural nails when working in the perinatal unit. When hands are not visibly soiled, alcohol-based hand hygiene products are effective in reducing microorganisms as long as the manufacturer's directions for use (DFU) are followed. Hand gels are also helpful because they are easier and quicker to use than hand washing and, therefore, help HCWs adhere to hand hygiene standards (Remington, Klein, Wilson, & Baker, 2006).

The Centers for Disease Control and Prevention (CDC) recommendation for standard precautions (see Chapter 1, "Basic Infection Control") and the Occupational Safety and Health Administration (OSHA) requirements need to be consistently followed in the area of perinatal care. Each newborn's bedside is considered its own separate clean environment, and as such, linens, instruments, and other items must not be shared between patients (Gilstrap & Oh, 2002). Perinatal HCWs should not perform routine care in other areas of the hospital in order to prevent transporting microorganisms into the perinatal area. If staff need to leave the area, surgical scrubs suits should be covered (Gilstrap & Oh, 2002).

With regard to vaginal deliveries, each personnel HCW assisting in the delivery must wear gowns, gloves, masks, and eye protection (Gilstrap & Oh, 2002). Gowns are not necessary for HCWs in the nursery as long as proper handwashing techniques are followed; however, gowns should be worn when holding the neonate outside the bassinet (Gilstrap & Oh, 2002). Operating room (OR) policies regarding all surgical procedures, including cesarean sections (C\S) must be followed. Gloves are always required for anyone coming into contact with blood or body secretions, for example, the newly delivered neonate prior to first bath, as well as the placenta. Strict sterile technique must be followed during all C\S, tubal ligations, or other sterile procedure, such as the placement of internal fetal electrodes or intrauterine pressure catheters (IUPC).

Neonatal linens and garments should be washed separately from other hospital laundry to prevent contamination and to retain softness (Gilstrap & Oh, 2002). All new linens and garments must be washed prior to neonatal use. All soiled linen need to be placed into impervious plastic hampers that can be easily disinfected and changed at least every 8 hours. Clean linens should be covered during transport into the nursery to prevent contamination. Gloved hands must be used when changing diapers to prevent contamination and prevent the spread of infection (Gilstrap & Oh, 2002; see Chapter 1, "Basic Infection Control" for gloving technique).

GENERAL DISCUSSION PUERPERAL INFECTION

Puerperal infection is generally used to describe any bacterial infection of the genital tract after delivery and is usually identified by a temperature of $38.0°C$ ($100.4°F$) or higher, occurring on any 2 of the first 10 days postpartum, exclusive of the first 24 hours (Cunningham et al., 2005, p. 712). Most fevers are caused by bacteria indigenous to the female genital tract, and this normal vaginal flora gets introduced during surgical procedures and contaminates wounds (Cunningham et al., 2005; Tharpe, 2008). Other sources of bacterial infection include surgical environment, HCWs, and instrument/supplies used during surgery. "With the advent of improved hygiene practices and the introduction of antibiotics, morbidity and mortality from puerperal infection had decreased significantly and infection is no longer the leading cause of maternal mortality" (Tharpe, 2008, p. 236).

The three main postoperative infections seen in C\S are endometritis, surgical site infection (SSI), and septic pelvic thrombophlebitis (SPT; Berghella, 2009). Endometritis, a localized infection at the placenta site or entire endometrium, is the most common cause of postpartum infection (Lowdermilk & Perry, 2004), with C\S being the most important risk factor for its development (Chen, 2008, p. 2). Women undergoing C\S delivery, especially those in labor prior to C\S, have an increased rate of puerperal fever and SSI compared with women undergoing vaginal deliveries (Tharpe, 2008). The pathogenesis of uterine infection with C\S is through infection of the surgical site; while for vaginal deliveries, it involves infection of the placental implantation site and surrounding tissue (Cunningham et al., 2005; Tharpe, 2008, p. 238).

PREVENTATIVE MEASURES

Preventative measures are the foundation of infection control, including hand washing and strict adherence to sterile technique, along with antibiotics use. Diligent evaluation of the patient's risk factors prior to delivery, along with consistent postpartum assessment, will allow for early detection of infection, enabling patients to receive prompt treatment.

There are a number of preventative measures for postpartum and postoperative infections. SSIs can occur as a result of C\S, laceration, or episiotomy (Berens, 2009). The three most critical aspects to prevent SSIs are general health of the patient, meticulous operative techniques, and preoperative antibiotics (Anderson & Sexton, 2008). Antibiotic use, typically given as a single perioperative dose, has been proven effective in decreasing infection (Cunningham et al., 2005, p. 712). Cephalosporins are the drugs of choice; however, clindamycin is often used in patients who are penicillin allergic (Tharpe, 2008). It is common practice to administer the drug at cord clamp so as not to mask any neonatal infection. However, research has shown that if the antibiotic was administered 15–50 minutes prior to procedure the risk of infection decreased without effecting neonatal outcomes (Berghella, 2009; Tharpe, 2008). Delay in antibiotic administration allows bacterial proliferation before therapeutic serum levels are reached (Tharpe, 2008). A second dose is recommended for surgery lasting more than 4 hours or with blood loss of more than 1500 ml (Meeks & Trenhaile, 2008).

Episiotomy is a surgical incision in the perineum performed at the time of delivery (Robinson, 2008). SSIs are usually seen in women with a midline episiotomy, 3rd or 4th degree laceration, or vaginal hematomas (Tharpe, 2008). Maintaining an intact perineum is extremely beneficial for infection prevention, especially in women with risk factors such as diabetes. Fever, tenderness, and discharge are common signs of an SSI that often occur 6–8 days postpartum. Most SSIs involving an episiotomy will heal with local perineal care (Robinson, 2008). Women who undergo vaginal deliveries are treated with similar preventative techniques except for limiting the number of vaginal exams and administering antibiotics in those women who are positive for Group B Streptococcal infections (discussed later in this chapter; Tharpe, 2008).

Many preoperative procedures have not been shown to reduce puerperal infections. For example, preoperative showering with 2% Chlorhexidine has shown to decrease microbial colony counts; however, it has not been shown to decrease SSIs (Anderson & Sexton, 2008; CDC, 1999). Similarly, preoperative hair removal is commonly performed before C/S, however, studies have shown that SSIs were highest among patients who shaved compared to clipping or the use of depilatory creams. The lowest risk of SSI was seen in patients leaving their hair intact (CDC, 1999; Tharpe, 2008). If hair needs to be removed, this should be done by clipping just prior to surgery as this has been shown to lower the risk of SSI compared with either shaving or clipping the night before (Anderson & Sexton, 2008; CDC, 1999). Patient skin preparation in the operating room usually consists of a preoperative wash using either povidone-iodine or chlorhexidine gluconate (CDC, 1999). Studies have not demonstrated a benefit (or harm) with skin cleaning, or an advantage of one antiseptic over another (Anderson & Sexton, 2008; Berghella, 2009). Vaginal antimicrobial preparations have not been shown to decrease the risk of fever, SSI, or endometritis; however, metronidazole gel has been shown to decrease postpartum endometritis. Drapes without adhesives appear to have lowed rates of wound infection (Berghella, 2009).

Finally, body temperature and tissue oxygenation impact the risk of SSIs (Meeks & Trenhaile, 2008). Maintaining perioperative normothermia can be accomplished through the use of warming blankets, along with putting booties and hats on patients (Anderson & Sexton 2008). Supplemental oxygen during and after surgeries has also been shown to reduce the risk of SSI and endometritis (Tharpe, 2008).

PREVENTATIVE MEASURES FOR OTHER DIAGNOSES

Fever in the puerperal period has a broad differential diagnosis (see Table 9.1). Atelectasis, alveolar collapse caused by hypoventilation, can be prevented by

TABLE 9.1

Causes of Fever in the Puerperal Period

Pelvic infection
Endometritis
SSI
Atelectasis
Septic pelvic thrombophlebitis
Urinary tract infection (UTI)
Mastitis
Complications of anesthesia

Adapted from Berens, 2009.

instructing patients to do coughing and deep breathing exercises postoperatively (Cunningham et al., 2005). Deep vein thrombosis (DVT), formation of a blood clot inside a blood vessel, occurs at a rate of 0.5 to 3 cases per 1,000 postpartum women (Lowdermilk & Perry, 2004). DVT can be prevented with the use of an automated pneumatic leg compression device and early ambulation (Berghella, 2009). Urethral catheterization is common prior to C/S to prevent distention of the bladder into the lower uterine segment; however, catheterization does increase the risk for UTI, another cause of puerperium fever. Even though some vaginal infections such as bacterial vaginosis and trichomonas vaginalis can be diagnosed ante partum, treatment of asymptomatic women has not been shown to prevent metritis (Cunningham et al., 2005).

Mastitis is a breast infection seen in about 1% of women after delivery (Lowdermilk & Perry, 2004). It presents as a unilateral, red, swollen, and tender area of one breast associated with fever. Patients also complain of chills, malaise, and flu-like symptoms. Women with a past history of mastitis, recent cracks or fissures around the nipple, use of a manual breast pump, and recent application of antifungal cream to the nipple area increase the risk of developing mastitis (Hopkinson & Schanler, 2009). Treatment requires supportive therapies in addition to antibiotics. Preventative measures include education on the signs and symptoms of mastitis and proper breastfeeding technique to avoid cracked nipples. Education is critical in this condition because mastitis usually occurs after discharge or about 1–4 weeks postpartum (Lowdermilk & Perry, 2004).

TORCH INFECTIONS AFFECTING NEWBORNS

TORCH is an acronym for toxoplasmosis, other infections (i.e., hepatitis, varicella), rubella virus, cytomegalovirus, and herpes simplex virus. Generally all TORCH infections produce flu-like symptoms for the mother, but are unfortunately associated with pregnancy and fetal complications (Lowdermilk & Perry, 2006).

Toxoplasmosis

Toxoplasmosis is caused by the protozoan *Toxoplasmosis gondii* (Lowdermilk & Perry, 2006). In the United States it is the third leading cause of death related to food-borne illnesses (CDC, 2008f). Although cats are the definitive host, the parasite is also found in sheep, cattle, dogs, and pigs (Lowdermilk & Perry, 2006). Most pregnant women contract the parasite by eating raw or undercooked meat or by contact with the feces of infected cats, either from the litter box or by gardening in areas where cats have defecated (Figure 9.1). Roughly one in three women who contract the disease during pregnancy pass the parasite onto their offspring. The chance of fetal infection ranges from 0.07% to 0.11% (Lowdermilk & Perry, 2006).

Toxoplasmosis increases the risk of miscarriage, stillbirths, premature delivery, neonatal death, and severe congenital anomalies (Olds, London, & Ladewig, 1992). Women are immune after the first episode unless immunocompromised (Lowdermilk & Perry, 2006). Symptoms can appear weeks, months, or even years

FIGURE 9.1

FIGURE 9.1

Cats are a definitive
parasite host for
Toxoplasmosis gondii

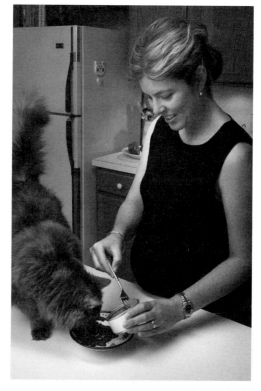

Courtesy of the Centers for Disease Control and Prevention. Photo by James Gathany.

after delivery, with complications ranging from mental disabilities to blindness and death (CDC, 2008f). Antimicrobial treatment of the pregnant mother reduces the infant's risk of becoming infected (Lowdermilk & Perry, 2006). Infants can also be treated with pyrimethamine, sulfadiazine, and folic acid if infected (Lowdermilk & Perry, 2006). However, the parasite may not be completely eliminated in pregnant women or infants as the parasite can remain in latent stages in certain tissues (CDC, 2008f). Preventative measures will reduce the risk of infection (see Table 9.2).

Syphilis

Syphilis is caused by a motile spirochete called *Treponema pallidum* and can be spread from mother to baby during delivery when coming in contact with the sore. Pregnancy effects include preterm labor, miscarriage, preterm birth, stillbirth, and congenital infection (Lowdermilk & Perry, 2006). Babies born to untreated pregnant women have a 40%–50% chance of showing signs of syphilis (Lowdermilk & Perry, 2006) (Figure 9.2). Prompt maternal treatment, usually with penicillin, reduces cases of congenital syphilis; however, treatment failure can occur, especially if treatment is given in the third trimester. Babies may be

TABLE **9.2**

Measures to Prevent Toxoplasmosis Infections

Avoid changing cat litter.
If you must change cat litter, wear gloves and wash your hands with soap and water immediately.
Change cat litter daily.
Feed your cat canned, not raw, food.
Avoid stray cats.
Keep your cat indoors.
Wear gloves while gardening.
Keep outside sand boxes covered.
Cook all food to safe cooking temperatures.
Peel and wash all fruits and vegetables.
Wash all utensils and cutting boards with hot soapy water.
Do not drink untreated water.
Freeze meat for several days prior to consumption.

From the Centers for Disease Control and Prevention, 2008f.

asymptomatic at birth; however, without immediate treatment they will, within weeks, develop major complications, including seizures, developmental delays, or death (CDC, 2008e). Even if the infant is treated early, adverse complications can occur later in life, such as neurosyphilis, deafness, joint involvement, and inflammation of the cornea (Lowdermilk & Perry, 2006) (Figure 9.3).

Women need to be tested for syphilis during the first prenatal visit and again in the third trimester if at high risk. However, false positives are not unusual, and one-third of people in the early primary stage will have negative test results (Lowdermilk & Perry, 2006). A positive test for syphilis must be reported to the board of health, and the patient needs to be offered HIV testing (CDC, 2008e).

Patients need to be instructed to abstain from sexual relations until treatment is complete, sores are gone, and serologic evidence of syphilis is proven negative. All sexual partners need to be contacted so they can be given treatment (CDC, 2008e). The only way to prevent syphilis is to abstain from sexual behavior or be involved in a mutual monogamous relationship with individuals who have documented negative results. Proper use of condoms can decrease your chance of contracting syphilis; however, condoms may be ineffective because the sore may be outside the area of condom sheathing. Certain techniques like douching, washing the genitals, urinating after intercourse, or using a condom with Nonoxynol-9, will not protect a person from syphilis (CDC, 2008e).

FIGURE **9.2**

Interstital keratitis related
to congenital syphilis

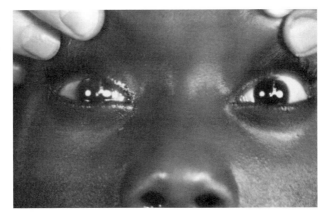

Courtesy of the Centers for Disease Control and Prevention / Susan Lindsley, VD.

FIGURE **9.3**

Congenital syphylis
facial lesion

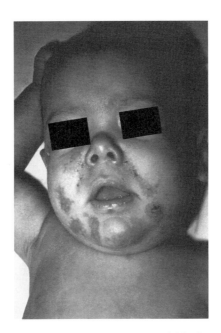

Courtesy of the Centers for Disease Control and Prevention / Dr. Joseph Caldwell.

Hepatitis B (HBV)

The most threatening virus to the newborn is the hepatitis B virus (HBV), which is a disease of the liver and is more contagious than HIV (Lowdermilk & Perry, 2006, p. 202). The CDC state that over 16,000 U.S. births each year are from hepatitis B surface antigen (HBsAg) positive women (Remington et al., 2006). Perinatal transmission occurs once the infant comes in contact with contaminated blood during delivery. Infants may contract perinatal HBV infection from highly infectious mothers; most of those infected will become chronic carriers and will be at increased risk for liver cirrhosis, liver cancer, and chronic hepatitis (Lowdermilk & Perry, 2006). Infants who develop overt hepatitis have a mortality rate of 75%. Women with HBV infection have a one in three chance of delivering preterm. Fetal malformation, intrauterine growth retardation (IUGR), and stillbirth are not associated with HBV infection (Lowdermilk & Perry, 2006).

Due to the severity of the disease and the availability of HBV vaccine and immunoglobulin (HBIG), the American Academy of Pediatrics (AAP) and the CDC recommend universal screening of all pregnant women for HBsAg during the first prenatal visit, and later in the pregnancy if the woman is at high risk (Lowdermilk & Perry, 2006; Remington et al., 2006). If testing was not done prior to hospital admission for delivery, or the patient is at high risk, HBsAg testing must be repeated (Gilstrap & Oh, 2002).

Vaccination should be offered to all newborns and all high-risk category women during pregnancy, including women with multiple sex partners, IV drug users, prostitutes, as well as women being treated for sexually transmitted infections (STIs). If infection is known at birth the infant should receive the HBV vaccine and HBIG within 12 hours, and then continue the vaccination series. With this prophylaxis, the chance of reducing perinatal infection is approximately 95% (Gilstrap & Oh, 2002).

Varicella

The varicella virus (VZV), which is responsible for the chickenpox and shingles, is a member of the herpes simplex family. The best way to prevent the disease is by vaccination prior to pregnancy. The risk of contracting the virus in pregnancy is low because the majority of women in their childbearing years are immune (Lowdermilk & Perry, 2006). However, contracting the virus during pregnancy can cause harmful effects to the fetus and a more severe case of VZV, including pneumonia, which has a mortality rate as high as 40% (Gilstrap & Oh, 2002).

Vertical transmission of the virus to the fetus during the first half of pregnancy can result in the congenital varicella syndrome (Pickering, 2006). One study reported the greatest risk for the development of congenital varicella syndrome is infection that occurs during the 13th to 20th week of pregnancy (CDC, 2007b). When VZV is contracted during the last 3 weeks of pregnancy approximately 25% of infants will develop clinical varicella (Lowdermilk & Perry, 2006.)

Women with VZV infection need airborne and contact precautions while hospitalized (Gilstrap & Oh, 2002). If the neonate contracts VZV they need to be kept isolated in a private room, adhering to airborne and contact precautions, for the duration of the illness. Neonates born to women with active VZV infection need to be kept isolated in the hospital for 21 days (if VZIG given) or 28 days (if VZIG not given; Gilstrap & Oh, 2002). Neonates, exposed postnatally should be isolated for 8–21 days (Gilstrap & Oh, 2002).

VZV vaccine is a live attenuated vaccine that cannot be given during pregnancy. Even though surveillance data has not shown any cases of fetal varicella syndrome after inadvertent exposures, a vaccinated woman should be educated to avoid pregnancy for 1 month (CDC, 2007b; Gilstrap & Oh, 2002). A child in the household of a pregnant woman can receive the VZV vaccine (Pickering, 2006). Prenatal screening should be done to discover the immune status of a woman; if nonimmune, the first dose of VZV vaccine should be given after delivery, with the second dose given 4–8 weeks later (Pickering, 2006). Vaccination is safe for the breastfeeding mother (CDC, 2007b). Preconception and prenatal screening and vaccination are the safest way to ensure the safety of mom and baby against VZV and its complications.

HIV TRANSMISSION FROM MOTHER TO BABY

When a baby is born to an HIV-infected woman the neonate has a 25% chance of contracting the disease if the woman has not received treatment (Gilstrap & Oh, 2002) (see Table 9.3). The primary mode of transmission is believed to be the infant's exposure to the mother's infected vaginal and cervical fluids (Lowdermilk & Perry, 2006). Breastfeeding for more than 12 months results in an additional 12%–14% of infants being infected (Lowdermilk & Perry, 2006). It is essential all women get counseling about the need for prenatal HIV testing as soon as possible in the pregnancy due to the dramatic decrease in perinatal transmission if proper intervention is begun. Since the access of antiviral prophylaxis (i.e., ZDV, AZT), the rate of perinatal transmission has been documented to be as low as 4% with vaginal delivery and as low as 2% if elective C/S is performed (Lowdermilk & Perry, 2006). With specific antiviral protocols in place, the Pediatric AIDS Clinical Trials Group (ACTG) Protocol 076 documented a 66% decrease in infant transmission (Lowdermilk & Perry, 2006; Remington et al., 2006).

Use standard precautions for HIV-positive women and infants. Because the mode of transmission appears to be delivery, it is recommended to promptly remove blood and body fluids from the infant immediately following delivery (Gilstrap & Oh, 2002). Breast milk contains the HIV virus; therefore, women need to be counseled not to breastfeed (Remington et al., 2006).

CHLAMYDIA

Chlamydia trachomatis is the most common sexually transmitted organism in the United States and may produce few to no symptoms (Pickering, 2006). It can cause irreversible damage to the reproductive organs, causing pelvic inflammatory

TABLE 9.3

Risk Factors for Neonatal HIV Transmission

Vaginal delivery
Ruptured membranes duration greater than 4 hours
Increased maternal viral load
Preterm birth
Multiple births
Duration of labor

Adapted from Lowdermilk & Perry, 2006.

disease (PID) and infertility. If exposed to HIV, these women are five times more likely to contract HIV (CDC, 2007a).

Chlamydia is contracted through vaginal, anal, or oral sex (CDC, 2007a). It can also be passed from mother to baby during delivery. The CDC recommends all women 25 years and younger, women with multiple or new sex partners, and women that do not use barrier methods be screened annually for chlamydia (CDC, 2007a). Universal screening of all pregnant women for chlamydia is recommended during the first prenatal visit and again in the third trimester if the woman is at high risk.

In pregnant women untreated chlamydia infections can lead to premature rupture of membranes and premature labor (CDC, 2007a; Lowdermilk & Perry, 2006). Babies who are born to chlamydia-infected women can get conjunctivitis (discussed later in this chapter) and pneumonia (CDC, 2007a). Because there is no prophylaxis for pneumonia, compared to conjunctivitis, babies at risk should get systemic antibiotics (Lowdermilk & Perry, 2006).

Maternal treatment includes a single dose of azithromycin or doxycycline 100 mg twice a day for 7 days (CDC, 2007a; Lowdermilk & Perry, 2006). All sex partners need to be treated to decrease the risk of reinfection. A repeat culture performed 3–4 months after treatment should be encouraged, especially if there is doubt regarding the treatment of their partner (CDC, 2007a).

The only way to prevent chlamydia is to abstain from sexual behavior or be involved in a mutual monogamous relationship with individuals who have documented negative results. To reduce the infection of chlamydia, latex condoms are helpful when used correctly (CDC, 2007a). The CDC recommends that anyone with possible signs or symptoms of an STI, such as urethral discharge, painful urination, or irregular bleeding, should abstain from sexual relations and seek medical care. Early treatment can prevent long term sequela. Infected women should tell all sex partners (within the last 60 days) to get tested (CDC, 2007a).

GONORRHEA

Gonorrhea is the oldest and one of the most common communicable diseases. It is aerobic, gram negative diplococcus that spreads almost entirely through sexual activity, usually through genital-to-genital contact (CDC, 2008g). Gonorrhea can be transmitted from mother to baby. Many men and women are asymptomatic, which is why screening needs to be done on the first prenatal visit and repeated in the third trimester if at high risk (Lowdermilk & Perry, 2006). Untreated gonorrhea can result in infertility (CDC, 2008g).

In pregnant women, gonorrhea can cause preterm labor, premature rupture of membranes, intra-amniotic infection, and miscarriage (Lowdermilk & Perry, 2006). Neonate complications include sepsis, joint infection, and conjunctivitis (Figure 9.4) (CDC, 2008g; Lowdermilk & Perry, 2006). Prevention of gonorrhea includes avoiding intercourse to avoid STIs and being in a monogamous relationship with an uninfected partner. Latex condoms decrease the risk for infection but will not eliminate it (CDC, 2008g).

Treatment requires patients to complete a course of antibiotics, abstain from intercourse, and return with any symptoms (CDC, 2008g). Infants who do contract

FIGURE 9.4

Neonatal complications of conjunctivitis from gonorrhea

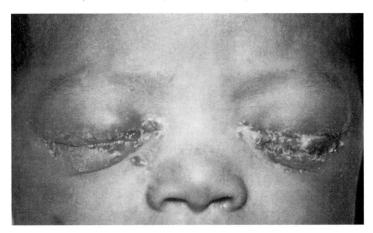

Courtesy of the Centers for Disease Control and Prevention / J. Pledger.

gonorrhea through passage of the infected birth canal rarely die from overwhelming infection, and neonates usually recover completely after appropriate treatment (Lowdermilk & Perry, 2006). Due to the increase in drug-resistant gonorrhea and the high possibility of the person being infected with other STIs, the CDC frequently updates their recommendations (CDC, 2008d; see http://www.cdc.gov). All cases of gonorrhea need to be reported to public health officials.

RUBELLA

Since rubella vaccination began in the late 1960s, cases of congenital rubella syndrome (CRS) have dramatically decreased (Lowdermilk & Perry, 2006), although outbreaks of rubella, also called the German measles, have been seen. Symptoms of rubella are not as severe for the mother as compared to the fetus (Figure 9.5). CRS can result in ophthalmologic, cardiac, auditory, and neurological problems (Pickering, 2006). The most severe abnormalities occur if the woman contracts the virus during the first trimester, with the risk of transmission to the infant being as high as 85%. This decreases to 54% during weeks 13–16, and then to 25% during the end of the second trimester (Lowdermilk & Perry, 2006; Pickering, 2006).

The virus can be cultured on infants for up to 18 months; therefore, it is mandatory that the infant be under extended pediatric droplet isolation until they are no longer contagious. Pharyngeal mucus and urine need to be free of the virus for the isolation precautions to be lifted (Lowdermilk & Perry, 2006).

The rubella vaccine is a live attenuated virus; therefore, it cannot be given during pregnancy. Women need to be counseled to avoid conception for 1 month due to possible teratogenic effects from the vaccine (Gilstrap & Oh, 2002; Pickering, 2006). If the vaccine is given inadvertently during pregnancy interruption

FIGURE **9.5**

"Blueberry muffin" skin
lesions of congenital
rubella

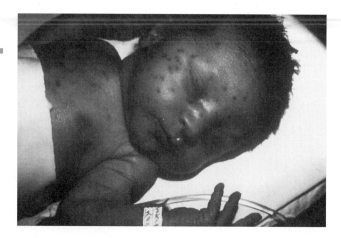

Courtesy of the Centers for Disease Control and Prevention.

of pregnancy is unnecessary because only signs of infection have been reported (Pickering, 2006). Breastfeeding is not a contraindication to the vaccine administration, so women should be offered the vaccine prior to being discharged from the hospital (Lowdermilk & Perry, 2006). A child in the home of a pregnant woman can be safely vaccinated; however, because the virus is shed in urine and other bodily fluids, it should not be given to someone who has close contact with an immunocompromised individual (Lowdermilk & Perry, 2006).

CYTOMEGALOVIRUS (CMV)

Cytomegalovirus (CMV) is the most common cause of viral infection in humans of all ages. It is a "silent" virus, meaning that the majority of people are asymptomatic or have flu-like symptoms. It is the most common virus transmitted from mother to baby (CDC, 2008a). Since 50%–80% of the population develops a CMV infection sometime before age 40, it is not surprising that 1% of newborns will contract CMV (CDC, 2008a; Lowdermilk & Parry, 2006). If a woman contracts CMV during pregnancy, the chance of spreading the disease to the infant is 1 in 3, but if the woman has a history of CMV infection, the chance decreases to 1 in 100 (CDC, 2008b). Most neonates are asymptomatic (approximately 90%) at birth; however, symptoms can appear later in life, such as hearing or vision loss and learning disabilities (Lowdermilk & Perry, 2006). CMV infection can cause miscarriage, stillbirth, or the more severe, congenital or neonatal cytomegalic inclusion disease (CMID; Lowdermilk & Perry, 2006). CMID is seen in approximately 1 in 150 babies, and approximately 1 in 750 children will develop permanent disabilities (CDC, 2008a).

Currently, there is no vaccine to prevent the disease or effective therapy for acute maternal infection; therefore, routine screening for the disease is ineffective (Gilstrap & Oh, 2002). However, certain steps can be taken to help prevent transmission of the virus.

CMV is spread by person-to-person contact (i.e., kissing, saliva, or sexual contact), breast milk, maternal fetal transmission, and blood transfusions (CDC,

2008c). The chance of getting CMV with causal contact is rare because people with previous CMV infections usually do not have the virus in body fluids, but you can contact CMV if active virus is present. "Contact with saliva and urine of young children is a major cause of CMV infection among pregnant women" (CDC, 2008c, p. 1). The best way to reduce the risk of CMV infection is proper hand washing. Other forms of protection are to limit contact with children's saliva and nasal secretions, disinfect surfaces that come into contact with any secretion, avoid sharing food and drinks with young children, and limit kissing children on the mouth or face (CDC, 2008a). The best way to prevent viral spread to the neonate is by educating pregnant women about proper hygienic practices.

HERPES SIMPLEX VIRUS (HSV)

Herpes simplex virus (HSV) is a widespread disease in the United States and infects one in five adolescents or adults. HSV causes genital ulcers that are painful and recurrent. HSV consists of two subtypes: HSV-1 (sexually transmitted) and HSV-2 (non–sexually transmitted, e.g., cold sores). However, each subtype is not exclusive (Lowdermilk & Perry, 2006). HSV is a recurrent and chronic disease with no known cure.

The highest risk of transmitting HSV to the newborn (33%–50%) occurs when the pregnant woman contracts a primary infection near the time of delivery, compared with the risk dropping significantly to less than 2%–5% if the infection is recurrent or if the woman contracted HSV during the first half of pregnancy (Figure 9.6) (CDC, 2008e; Gilstrap & Oh, 2002). Women who contract primary HSV infection during pregnancy have an increased risk of miscarriage (Lowdermilk & Perry, 2006), preterm birth, and IUGR (uptodate, HSV, 2009). The worst complication with HSV is neonatal herpes ,which has a 60% infant mortality rate, and half of those infants that survive have serious neurologic complications (Lowdermilk & Perry, 2006).

Obstetric management for genital HSV requires careful questioning and examination of the women upon admission to the hospital. The CDC and ACOG have specific recommendations about when a patient can deliver vaginally or via C/S, along with recommendations for treating with antiviral therapy, such as acyclovir, to decrease risk of transmission of HSV to the infant (Gilstrap & Oh, 2002). Two main things should be considered with the decision to treat the patient with antiviral therapy. First is the timing of infection relative to delivery, and second is the category of infection—primary vs. recurrent (CDC, 2009). Acyclovir has been proven to decrease HSV outbreak at time of delivery, decrease viral shedding and decrease C/S rates (uptodate, HSV, February 2009).

Standard precautions are sufficient in dealing with HSV infection, and regular cleaning of the labor and delivery room is sufficient to disinfect a hospital room (Gilstrap & Oh, 2002). Contact precautions are necessary in regards to caring for a patient with an active HSV infection (Gilstrap & Oh, 2002). Babies born vaginally to women with active lesions should be placed in contact isolation and physically separated from other infants in the nursery. An isolation room is not critical (Gilstrap & Oh, 2002). Standard precautions are used for the neonate born to women with recurrent disease who do not have active lesions and were

FIGURE **9.6**

Herpes simplex skin
lesions

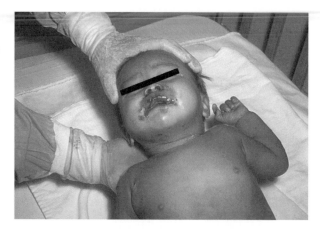

Courtesy of the Centers for Disease Control and Prevention / J. D. Millar.

delivered via C/S. An infant with positive cultures, with or without symptoms, needs to be in an isolation room and managed with contact precautions for the duration of the illness. Gowns and gloves should be used with any HCW who has skin lesions or potentially infectious secretions (Gilstrap & Oh, 2002).

Careful hand washing is critical to prevention. All infected women need to be taught about hygienic measures to prevent transmission to the baby (Gilstrap & Oh, 2002). The women should be educated to wash hands thoroughly and use a clean barrier to ensure that the baby does not come into contact with any lesions. A women with HSV 2 (cold sores) needs to be told not to kiss or snuggle with her baby to prevent infection until the lesions have cleared (Gilstrap & Oh, 2002). The mother can wear a mask to help prevent accidental touching of an active lesion. All family members with active lesions need also to be educated on how to keep the baby HSV free (Gilstrap & Oh, 2002).

Education is important for couples dealing with HSV. Education should include potential for recurrent episodes, asymptomatic viral shedding, and sexual transmission (CDC, 2009). HCWs must stress that viral shedding can take place even when patients are asymptomatic, and contraction of HSV can take place at any time. Couples need to be told not to have sexual contact if they have or suspect an HSV outbreak. The CDC advises pregnant women to avoid sexual contact during the third trimester with men who have HSV (CDC, 2009). Proper use of condoms will decrease but not eliminate the chance of contracting HSV. Prevention of neonatal herpes depends on avoiding HSV infection during the late stages of pregnancy and avoiding infant contact with lesions at the time of delivery (CDC, 2009).

PREVENTATIVE CARE MEASUREJS FOR THE INFANT

Eye Infection Prophylaxis

In the United States it is mandatory that all neonates, whether delivered via vaginal or C/S, receive instillation of a prophylactic agent in the eyes to protect against ophthalmia neonatorum (Lowdermilk & Perry, 2004). These antimicrobial agents are given to provide protection against *Neisseria gonorrhea* and *Chlamydia trachomatis* (Lowdermilk & Perry, 2004). As the newborn passes through the infected birth canal, gonorrheal or chlamydial infections can be contracted by the infant, causing an inflammation of the newborn's eye (Remington et al., 2006). Without treatment the gonococcal eye infection can cause corneal scarring or blindness; however, the risk of severe ocular damage from a chlamydia eye infection is low (Remington et al., 2006). Treatment of ophthalmia neonatorum is primarily for the prevention of the more severe gonococcal sequelae (Remington et al., 2006).

Eye prophylaxis consists of administering antimicrobials as soon after birth as possible; however, some hospital protocols allow it to be given within 1 hour after birth to help parent–infant attachment. After cleaning the infant's eyelids, the antimicrobial agent should be administered directly into the conjunctival sac by applying a 1- to 2-centimeter ribbon. The agent used for prophylaxis varies by institution; however, current recommendations from the CDC include aqueous silver nitrate 1%, erythromycin ophthalmic ointment 0.5%, or tetracycline ophthalmic ointment 1% (Cunningham et al., 2005). Silver nitrate is not effective against chlamydia and has a 50% chance of causing chemical conjunctivitis (Remington et al., 2006). In developed countries erythromycin and tetracycline are more widely used, whereas developing countries use silver nitrate (which is readily available and inexpensive), given its effectiveness in areas where penicillinase-producing gonococcal infections are endemic (Remington et al., 2006).

Omphalitis

Umbilical cord care is extremely important to help prevent an umbilical infection known as omphalitis. After birth, the umbilical cord tissue remnant slowly dies and ultimately falls off. This necrotic tissue mass serves as an outstanding media for bacterial growth and infection. Because the umbilical cord is in close proximity to the umbilical vessels, bacteria can have direct access to the bloodstream. One should care for an umbilical cord as one would care for a wound infection. Bacterial colonization is reduced by the application of topical antimicrobial agents. During each diaper change, the HCW should assess the umbilical cord site in order to monitor edema, redness, and purulent discharge (Lowdermilk & Perry, 2004). The cord clamp, which is placed on at delivery, should be removed when the cord is dry, approximately 24 hours later.

Summary of Group B Streptococcus (GBS)

Group B streptococcus (GBS) may be considered part of the normal vaginal transient flora of women, pregnant or not pregnant; however, it continues to cause serious neonatal infection (CDC, 2002). The human reservoir for GBS is the gastrointestinal tract, which leads to vaginal colonization. Ten to 30% of pregnant women are colonized with GBS (CDC, 2002). Prenatal screening identifies intrapartum GBS colonization and decreases vertical transmission from infected mother to the infant during delivery (see Figure 9.7).

FIGURE **9.7**

CDC algorithm for GBS intrapartum chemoprophylaxis

Indications for intrapartum antibiotic prophylaxis to prevent perinatal GBS disease under a universal prenatal screening strategy based on combined vaginal and rectal cultures collected at 37–37 weeks' gestation from all pregnant women

Vaginal and rectal GBS screening cultures at 35–37 weeks' gestation for **ALL** pregnant women (unless patient had GBS bacteriuria during the current pregnancy or a previous infant with invasive GBS disease)

Intrapartum prophylaxis indicated	**Intrapartum prophylaxis not indicated**

• Previous infant with invasive GBS disease
 	
• GBS bacteriuria during current pregnancy
 	
• Positive GBS screening culture during current pregnancy (unless a planned cesarean delivery, in the absence of labor or amniotic membrane rupture, is performed)
 	
• Unknown GBS status (culture not done, incomplete, or results unknown) and any of the following:
  • Delivery at <37 weeks' gestation*
  • Amniotic membrane rupture > 18 hours
  • IIntrapartum temperature > 100.4˚F (>38.0˚C)†
	• Previous pregnancy with a positive GBS screening culture (unless a culture was also positive during the current pregnancy)
	
	• Planned cesarean delivery performed in the absence of labor or membrane rupture (regardless of maternal GBS culture status)
	
	• Negative vaginal and rectal GBS screening culture in late gestation during the current pregnancy, regardless of intrapartium risk factors

From the Centers for Disease Control and Prevention, MMWR, August 16, 2002.

* If onset of labor or rupture of amniotic membranes occurs at <37 weeks' gestation and there is a significant risk for preterm delivery (as assessed by the clinician), a suggested algorithm for GBS prophylaxis management is provided.

† If amnionitis is suspected, broad-spectrum antibiotic therapy that includes an agent known to be active against GBS should replace GBS Prophylaxis.

Although GBS can cause maternal complications, such as UTIs, chorioamnionitis, endometritis, sepsis, and wound infections, most women are asymptomatic (Ransom, Dombrowski, Evans, & Ginsburg, 2002, p. 147). Maternal death from GBS-associated infections is extremely rare (CDC, 2002).

Risk Factors for Neonatal GBS Disease

- Positive GBS culture with the current pregnancy
- Intrapartum fever with temperature above 100.4°F
- Premature rupture of membranes more than 18 hours before delivery
- Premature delivery earlier than 37 weeks
- Low birth weight
- Positive history for early onset neonatal GBS (Lowdermilk & Perry, 2004, pp. 209, 1069)

Fetal infection occurs either by aspiration of infected amniotic fluid or during passage through the birth canal. Fetal aspiration of GBS-infected amniotic fluid can lead to neonatal pneumonia, stillbirth, or sepsis. Vaginal transmission during delivery results in GBS colonization of the skin or mucous membranes and is usually asymptomatic (CDC, 2002).

GBS disease in infants is classified into early or late onset. Early onset disease is usually seen in infants younger than 7 days of age and generally within the first 24 hours of life (Pickering, 2006). Clinical manifestation of early onset disease include systemic infection, respiratory distress, pneumonia, and, less common, meningitis (Pickering, 2006). Late onset disease occurs in infants between the ages of 1 week and 3 months and commonly manifests as an occult bacteremia with focal infection, such as meningitis, osteomyelitis, or septic arthritis (Pickering, 2006, p. 621).

The most effective way to reduce GBS disease is proper screening with a bacterial vaginal/rectal culture on selective broth media between 35–37 weeks of pregnancy and treatment with intrapartum chemoprophylaxis, which has been shown to reduce the risk of GBS disease. Antepartum chemoprophylaxis does not eradicate the disease, and postpartum (neonatal) chemoprophylaxis has not been shown to reduce the incidence of early or late onset GBS disease (Ransom et al., 2002).

POST-TEST QUESTIONS

9-1. One of the main post-operative infections seen after caesarean section surgery is:
   a. Endometritis
   b. Episiotomy infection
   c. Hepatitis B infection
   d. Chlamydia infection

9-2. Which of the following describes a breast infection?
   a. Toxoplasmosis
   b. Thrombophlebitis
   c. Atelectasis
   d. Mastitis

9-3. Which of the following organisms can cause eye infections in the neonate if routine eye infection prophylaxis is not administered?
   a. Group B streptococcus
   b. *Neiserria gonorrhea*

    c. Herpes simplex virus

    d. Cytomegalovirus

9-4. TORCH is an acronym for:

    a. Tularemia, other infections, rickettsia, cytomegalovirus, herpes simplex virus

    b. Tularemia, other infections, rubella, Chlamydia, herpes simplex virus

    c. Toxoplasmosis, other infections, rubella, cytomegalovirus, herpes simplex virus

    d. Toxoplasmosis, other infections, rubella, cytomegalovirus, herpes zoster virus

9-5. All of the following are vaccine-preventable illnesses that can spread to the neonate during pregnancy or during delivery *except*:

    a. Chlamydia

    b. Rubella

    c. Varicella

    d. Hepatitis B

References

Centers for Disease Control and Prevention. (1999). *Guideline for prevention of surgical site infection, 1999.* Retrieved August 1, 2009, from CDC Web site.

Centers for Disease Control and Prevention. (2002). Prevention of perinatal group streptococcal disease: Revised guidelines from the CDC. *MMWR, 51* (RR11), 1–22. Retrieved January 1, 2009, from http://www.cdc.gov/mmwr/preview/mmwrhtml/rr5111a1.htm

Centers for Disease Control and Prevention. (December 20, 2007a). *Chlamydia CDC fact sheet.* Retrieved January 9, 2009, from http://www.cdc.gov/std/chlamydia/STDFact-2006Chlamydia.htm

Centers for Disease Control and Prevention. (June 12, 2007b). *Vaccines & preventable disease: Varicella vaccine-Q&As about pregnancy.* Retrieved January 2, 2009, from http://www.cdc.gov/vaccines/vpd-vac/varicella/vac-faqs-clinic-preg.htm

Centers for Disease Control and Prevention. (2008a). *About CMV.* Retrieved January 3, 2009, from http://www.cdc.gov/cmv/facts.htm

Centers for Disease Control and Prevention. (2008b). *CDC features: Learn about cytomegalovirus.* Retrieved January 3, 2009, from http://www.cdc.gov/Features/Cytomegalovirus/

Centers for Disease Control and Prevention. (2008c). *Frequently asked questions about CMV.* Retrieved January 3, 2009, from http://www.cdc.gov/cmv/faqs.htm

Centers for Disease Control and Prevention. (2008d). *Gonorrhea CDC fact sheet.* Retrieved January 5, 2009, from http://www.cdc.gov/std/Gonorrhea/STDFact-gonorrhea.htm

Centers for Disease Control and Prevention. (2008e). *Syphilis: CDC fact sheet.* Retrieved January 10, 2009, from http://www.cdc.gov/std/syphilis/STDFact-Syphilis.htm

Centers for Disease Control and Prevention. (2008f). *Toxoplasmosis.* Retrieved January 10, 2009, from http://www.cdc.gov/toxoplasmosis/index.html

Centers for Disease Control and Prevention. (2008g). *Updated recommended treatment options for gonoccal infections and associated conditions-United States April 2007.* Retrieved January 5, 2009, from http://www.cdc.gov/STD/treatment/2006/updated-regimens.htm

Centers for Disease Control and Prevention. (2009). *Genital herpes simplex (HSV) module.* Retrieved July 25, 2009, from www2a.cdc.gov/stdtraining/ready-to-use/Manuals/HSV/hsv-notes-2009.doc

Anderson, D.J., & Sexton, A.J. (2008). *Control measures to prevent surgical site infection.* Retrieved July 15, 2009, from http://uptodate.com

Berghella, V. (2009). *Cesarean delivery: Preoperative Issues.* Retrieved July 15, 2009, from http://uptodate.com

Berens, P. (2009). *Overview of postpartum care.* Retrieved July 15, 2009, from http://uptodate.com

Chen, K.T. (2008). *Postpartum endometritis.* Retrieved July 7, 2009, from http://uptodate.com

Cunningham, F.G., Hauth, J.C., Leveno, K.J., Gilstrap, L., Bloom, S.L., & Wenstrom, K.D. (2005). *Williams obstetrics* (22nd ed.). New York: McGraw-Hill.

Gilstrap, L.C., & Oh, W. (2002). *Guidelines for perinatal care* (5th ed.). Elk Grove Village, IL: American Academy for Pediatrics and the American College of Obstetricians and Gynecologists.

Hopkinson, J. & Schanler, R. J. (2009). Common problems of breastfeeding in the postpartum period. Retrieved July 15, 2009, from http://uptodateonline.com/online/content/topic.do?topicKey=neonatol/21625&view=print

Lowdermilk, D. L, & Perry, S.E. (2004). *Maternity and women's health care* (8th ed.). St. Louis, MO: Mosby.

Lowdermilk, D. L., & Perry, S. E. (2006). Maternity Nursing. (7th ed.) St. Louis, MO: Mosby.

Meeks, G.R., & Trenhaile, T. (2008). *Abdominal surgical incisions: Prevention and treatment of complications.* Retrieved July 15, 2009, from http://uptodate.com

Olds, S.B., London, M.L. & Ladewig, P. W. (1992). Maternal Newborn Nursing (4th edition). Redwood, CA: Addison-Wesley Nursing.

Pickering, L.K. (2006). *Red book: 2006 report of the Committee of Infectious Diseases* (27th ed.). Elk Grove Village, IL: American Academy of Pediatrics.

Ransom, S.B., Dombrowski, M.P., Evans, M.I., & Ginsburg, K.A. (2002). *Contemporary therapy in obstetrics and gynecology.* Philadelphia: W.B. Saunders Company.

Remington, J.S., Klein, J.O., Wilson, C.B., & Baker, C.J. (2006). *Infectious disease of the fetus and newborn infant.* Philadelphia: Saunders.

Robinson, J.N. (2008). *Approach to episiotomy.* Retrieved July 15, 2009, from http://uptodate.com

Tharpe, N. (2008). Postpregnancy genital tract and wound infections. *Journal of Midwifery and Women's Health, 53*(May/June).

Infection Control in Dialysis

10

This chapter includes topics on the methods of infection prevention in a dialysis center. The causative organisms and treatment options are reviewed. There is discussion on end-stage renal disease and equipment disinfection measures specific to this specialty area.

OBJECTIVES

1. Define the members and role of the infection prevention committee.
2. Delineate the components of an infection prevention plan.
3. Identify methods of infection prevention in a dialysis center.
4. Identify causative organisms and treatments.
5. Identify infection prevention specific to dialysis.

PRE-TEST QUESTIONS

10-1. In a dialysis unit, gloves should be worn:
   a. When performing routine tasks (i.e., answering the phone)
   b. When walking around the unit
   c. When performing aseptic procedures
   d. When touching "clean" equipment

10-2. A dialysis machine should be internally cleaned with bleach after it has been used to dialyze a patient with:
   a. Hepatitis B infection
   b. An upper respiratory tract infection
   c. Influenza infection
   d. Methicillin-sensitive *S. Aureus* infection

10-3. All of the following are necessary to prevent transmission of infection *except*:
   a. Hand washing
   b. Gloving
   c. Proper disposal of waste products
   d. Routine use of prophylactic antibiotics

10-4. To disinfect the external surfaces of nondisposable equipment in a dialysis unit, which of the following should be used?
   a. 1:100 bleach solution
   b. 1:100 vinegar solution
   c. 1:100 isopropyl alcohol solution
   d. 1:100 hydrochloric acid solution

10-5. Routine precautions for the care of the hemodialysis patient recommended by the CDC include:
   a. Patients should have specific dialysis stations assigned to them.
   b. Nondisposable items (such as chairs, etc.) must be cleaned at the end of each day.
   c. Medications should be prepared on a central medication cart and then taken to the patient's bedside.
   d. Clean and contaminated areas can be in the same area as long as they are clearly marked.

Infection prevention among chronic hemodialysis patients is an area that has recently undergone intense scrutiny from the Centers for Medicare and Medicaid (CMS). As the largest monetary supporter of end stage renal disease (ESRD) patients, CMS has the authority to mandate regulations that must be followed by hemodialysis centers. These regulations are instituted by CMS and are delegated to the local state authority for enforcement (Department of Health and Human Services, Centers for Medicare and Medicaid Services, 2008)

The initial step in ensuring prevention of the spread of infection in a dialysis unit is the development of an infection prevention committee. This committee should minimally include an infection control–certified nurse, the medical director of the dialysis center, nurse manager of the dialysis center, and a member from the technical department of the dialysis center. Other members may include other members of the interdisciplinary team, such as the social worker or dietitian.

The infection prevention committee is charged with developing policies and audit tools as well as monitoring the dialysis unit for breaches in infection prevention. Monitoring of infections is also an integral part of identifying and addressing issues in order to decrease the chance for the spread of infection.

Before embarking on enforcing infection prevention practices, it is important to establish a game plan. Planning begins with outlining, in policy form, the guidelines that staff must follow. The guidelines should include the items in Table 10.1.

All policies and guidelines should be reviewed periodically and updated to reflect changes in regulations and Centers for Disease Control and Prevention (CDC) guidelines.

TABLE 10.1
Dialysis Facility Guidelines for Infection Control

- Standard precautions including personal protective equipment (PPE).
- When, how often, and for how long hands should be washed.
- Gloving procedures.
- Standards for disinfection of equipment.
- Proper handling and disposal of infectious or potentially infectious material, that is, regulated versus nonregulated waste.
- Health care worker (HCW) dress code.
- HCW screening and vaccines offered.
- When and where food and drink may be ingested by HCWs and patients.
- Housekeeping policy and schedule.

STANDARD PRECAUTIONS

Initially called *universal precautions,* standard precaution is the act of treating *all* patients as if they are actively infected with bloodborne pathogens (Siegel, Rhinehart, Jackson, Chiarello, & the Healthcare Infection Control Practices Advisory Committee, 2007). This includes the items in Table 10.2.

TABLE 10.2
Standard Precautions in a Dialysis Facility

- The use of PPE when there is the possibility of exposure to blood or body fluids.
- Cleaning up spills of blood and/or other infectious materials with an appropriate disinfectant immediately.
- Immediately changing scrubs or clothes that become soiled with blood or body fluids.
- No visitors in the dialysis unit during initiation and discontinuation of treatment.
- No eating, drinking, smoking, applying cosmetics, or applying lip balm by patients or HCWs in the dialysis unit.
- No bare feet in the unit.
- PPE must never be worn outside the patient care area (i.e., waiting room).
  - PPE includes mask, shield, gloves, and an impermeable gown.

According to the CDC, hand washing is the single most important means of preventing the spread of infection (Figure 10.1) (see Chapter 1, "Basic Infection Control"). As early as 1843, Dr. Oliver Wendell Holmes advocated hand washing to prevent child bed fever (Case, n.d.). Hands must be washed thoroughly and often (Table 10.3). Wash hands for a minimum of 15 seconds, scrubbing between fingers, the backs of hands, and around thumbs. Hands should be completely dried after washing. For the complete procedure for correct hand-washing technique, see Chapter 1, "Basic Infection Control" (CDC, 2001). Hand washing should be monitored by a person assigned to infection prevention monitoring. Noncompliance with unit policy should be documented and reported at the infection prevention meeting. HCWs in violation of the policy should be reeducated or disciplined based on severity of the violation.

HCWs and patients alike are frequently unaware of the many instances where a breach in infection prevention practice has occurred. It is a mistaken perception that gloves can replace washing your hands. Gloves will protect the wearer, but not necessarily anyone else. As soon as the person wearing the gloves touches anything, the gloves become contaminated and can then be a vector for infection transmission.

Gloving

Gloves are an important part of infection prevention; however, they must be used correctly (see Table 10.4). Gloves should be worn to protect the patient and the caregiver. Gloves *do not* take the place of effective, appropriate hand washing. For a complete discussion on the correct procedures for open-gloving and closed-gloving, see Chapter 1.

Disinfection of Equipment

Nondisposable equipment used in the dialysis facility must be disinfected frequently. Minimally, this is done between each patient. The area where the patient receives treatment "belongs" to that patient until they leave the unit. The area

FIGURE 10.1

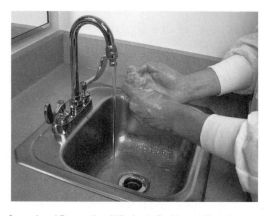

Courtesy of the Centers for Disease Control and Prevention / Kimberly Smith and Christine Ford. Photo by Kimberly Smith.

TABLE 10.3

Hand Washing Requirements in a Dialysis Facility

IN A DIALYSIS UNIT HANDS MUST BE WASHED

- When entering the unit.
- Whenever contact may be made with blood or body fluids.
- After removal of gloves.
- Before reaching into a box for gloves or supplies.
- After contact with machines.
- After sneezing or blowing your nose.
- After use of the restroom.
- After eating.
- When leaving the unit.

---

is considered dirty while the patient is there. Surface disinfection may only be initiated when the patient completes his or her treatment and physically leaves the area. Using separate, disposable, single-use cloths for the machine, chair, and television (where applicable), a cloth soaked with a 1:100 bleach solution should be utilized to wipe all external surfaces. *All* areas must be properly cleansed to prevent the spread of bloodborne pathogens. New disposable equipment cannot be brought into the treatment area until the patient has left and the area has been disinfected.

All equipment must be surface cleaned. This includes anything brought into the patient area, such as a medication pump. Check the manufacturer's directions for use (DFU) and the facility policy to ensure compliance is maintained. The hemodialysis machine must undergo routine disinfection according to the manufacturer's DFU (for a picture of a dialysis machine, see Figure 10.2). All hemodialysis machines are supplied with recommendations and instructions from the manufacturer regarding proper disinfection. It is the responsibility of the dialysis facility management to ensure staff is educated on these guidelines and abides by them.

Hemodialysis Machine Disinfection

1. Daily disinfection with vinegar and heat unless bleach is used.
2. Twice weekly disinfection with bleach after vinegar, without heat cycle.
3. Bleach disinfection after dialyzer blood leak.
4. Bleach disinfection after patients with active infections such as:
   a. Hepatitis B virus (HBV)
   b. Methicillin-resistant *Staphylococcus aureus* (MRSA)
   c. Vancomycin-resistant enterococcus (VRE)
5. Bleach disinfection after repairs.

TABLE **10.4**

Correct Glove Use

GLOVES SHOULD BE WORN

▓ Whenever the potential for exposure to blood and /or body fluids is present.

▓ When performing tasks on "contaminated or dirty" equipment.

▓ When performing aseptic procedures.

GLOVES SHOULD *NOT* BE WORN

▓ When performing routine tasks (i.e., answering the phone).

▓ When walking around the dialysis unit.

▓ When leaving the dialysis unit.

▓ When touching "clean" equipment.

▓ During routine patient care, such as taking blood pressure.

GLOVES *MUST* BE CHANGED

▓ Between patients.

▓ When visibly soiled.

▓ When going from dirty to clean area.

Regulated Medical Waste

The definition of *regulated medical waste* (RMW) is any solid waste generated in the diagnosis, treatment, or immunization of human beings and includes human blood and blood products, as well as sharps (New Jersey Administrative Code, n.d.). All waste that is considered regulated is collected in segregated trash cans with red liner bags (see Figures 10.3–10.5). The containers must be rigid, leak-resistant, impervious to moisture, sufficiently strong to prevent tearing or bursting under normal circumstances, and sealed to prevent leakage during transport.

RMW is collected by companies licensed in Hazardous Materials for transport and destruction (see Chapter 11, "Medical Waste Disposal"). RMW has a cost associated with it as the facility is charged either by weight or by container volume. The facility must seal and label all containers prior to pick up. It is the HCWs responsibility to segregate regular trash from RMW and to take care when discarding items. Nonregulated medical waste (paper, plastic, etc.) can be discarded in the regular trash per unit policy. (See Chapter 11 for a complete discussion of regulated medical waste.)

Infections

The number of patients with ESRD increases each year. These patients require some form of renal replacement therapy (i.e., hemodialysis, peritoneal dialysis, or

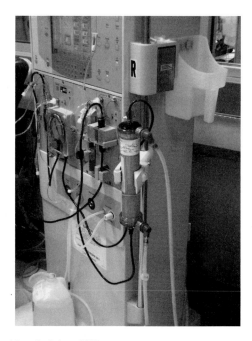

FIGURE 10.2

Dialysis machine

Photograph used with permission of Amelia Gajary, 2010

renal transplantation) to sustain life. The number of hemodialysis patients alone has increased dramatically. Because of the nature and treatment of their disease, hemodialysis patients are at a high risk for infection. Consequently, there are definitive recommendations to prevent infections (see Tables 10.5 and 10.6). While already immunocompromised by kidney disease, these patients

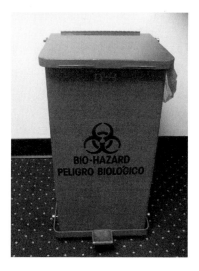

FIGURE 10.3

Biohazard container

Photograph used with permission of Amelia Gajary, 2010.

FIGURE **10.4**

Red liner bag

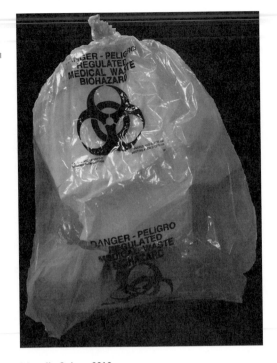

Photograph used with permission of Amelia Gajary, 2010.

FIGURE **10.5**

Biohazard container

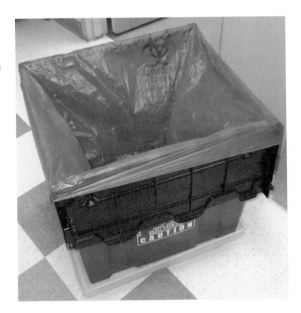

Photograph used with permission of Amelia Gajary, 2010.

are exposed to potential infections that may occur as a result of the vascular access that is used for dialysis. The hemodialysis access is used up to three times a week for several hours each treatment. For patients receiving in-center hemodialysis, this occurs in an area where other patients are being treated simultaneously. Additionally, the patient to caregiver ratio (typically 3:1) exposes the patient to a greater risk of person-to-person transmission of infection. Aseptic technique must be maintained whenever the possibility of transmitting infectious agents is possible (see Chapter 1, "Basic Infection Control"). Hand washing, gloving, proper disinfection, and proper disposal of waste products are essential ingredients in preventing infection. It is up to the HCW to maintain good habits to prevent infection in the vascular access.

There are several types of infections that are of concern in the hemodialysis unit. HBV was of major concern in the 1970s and 1980s. This is a bloodborne pathogen that can live for up to 10 days on a surface that is not appropriately disinfected. The incidence of HBV infections has diminished greatly over the years, in large part due to the successful vaccine immunization program of patients and staff against the virus. The vaccine is administered to patients as a series of doses given over a 6-month period. Immunocompromised patients such as those receiving dialysis should receive a series of four injections at months 0, 1, 2, and 6. HCWs and those who are not immunocompromised should receive a series of three injections at months 0, 1, and 6 (see Chapter 3, "Immunizations"). It is vitally important that HCWs and patients receive these immunizations. It is the role of the HCW to educate patients on the importance of protecting themselves against this potentially lethal virus.

Hepatitis C virus (HCV) has become somewhat prevalent in the dialysis population. Due to the rise in the number of cases of this strain of hepatitis, the CDC

TABLE 10.5

CDC Recommended Precautions to Minimize the Risk for Infection in Hemodialysis Patients

- Patients should have specific dialysis stations assigned to them.
- Nondisposable items (such as chairs, etc.) must be cleaned after each use.
- *No* sharing of nondisposable items if possible. Items that are shared (i.e., BP cuffs) must be disinfected after each use.
- Medications and supplies should not be shared and medication carts should *not be used.*
- Medications should be prepared and distributed from a centralized area.
- Clean and contaminated areas should be separated
  - within the treatment area (clean sinks for hand washing versus dirty sinks for draining saline bags and other fluid)
  - outside of the treatment area (clean and dirty utility rooms)
- Standard precautions must be maintained.

TABLE 10.6

System Controls to Prevent Dialysis Infections

- Optimize the resistance of the patient to infection. (Vaccinate, practice good infection prevention.)
- Control reservoir of infections. (Separate infected persons.)
- Limit transmission of infectious agents. (Follow infection prevention guidelines.)
- Maintain local defenses: intact skin. (Cleanse appropriately and monitor integrity.)
- Improve/provide specific immunity. (Immunizations.)
- Optimize treatment of underlying diseases such as diabetes mellitus to improve resistance. (Report to the nephrologist any changes in patient condition for referral to their primary medical practitioner.)

formulated recommendations for the prevention and control of HCV infection and HCV-related disease. (CDC, 1998).

Bacterial Infections

Bacterial infections are also of concern. With the increasing use of antibiotics over the recent past, bacteria have mutated, and multidrug-resistant organisms (MDROs) have become much more common. Two such bacterial infections are methicillin-resistant *Staphylococcus aureus* (MRSA) and vancomycin-resistant enterococcus (VRE). Due to these MDROs, the judicious use of antibiotics is paramount. Whenever possible, blood cultures with sensitivity testing should be obtained to identify possible bloodstream infection (BSI). It is important that facility HCWs perform timely monitoring of lab testing results and communicate these findings to the physician for appropriate antibiotic adjustment.

Miscellaneous Issues

HCWs are advised to wear scrubs and dedicated shoes when caring for hemodialysis patients. Ideally, scrubs should be removed prior to leaving the dialysis facility; however, if this is not feasible, they should be removed as soon as the employee arrives home. Scrubs should never be worn outside of the workplace as they may spread potentially infectious microorganisms into the community. Soiled scrubs should be removed immediately.

All units should have a post-exposure prophylaxis (PEP) policy in the event a HCW is injured by contact with blood or body fluid or by needlestick (Figure 10.6). It is important that all HCWs know the policy and whom to contact in the event of an exposure. It is in the HCW's best interest to report exposures immediately to minimize their risk. *Remember, infection prevention begins with you. Hand washing, aseptic technique, good hygiene, and personal responsibility are important tools in infection prevention, but you are the most important component in making it work.*

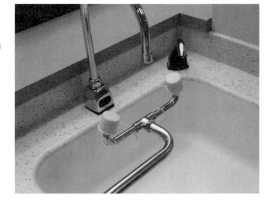

FIGURE 10.6

Eye wash

Photograph used with permission of Amelia Gajary, 2010.

POST-TEST QUESTIONS

10-1. In a dialysis unit, gloves should be worn:
   a. When performing routine tasks (i.e., answering the phone)
   b. When walking around the unit
   c. When performing aseptic procedures
   d. When touching "clean" equipment

10-2. A dialysis machine should be internally cleaned with bleach after it has been used to dialyze a patient with:
   a. Hepatitis B infection
   b. An upper respiratory tract infection
   c. Influenza infection
   d. Methicillin-sensitive *S. Aureus* infection

10-3. All of the following are necessary to prevent transmission of infection *except*:
   a. Hand washing
   b. Gloving
   c. Proper disposal of waste products
   d. Routine use of prophylactic antibiotics

10-4. To disinfect the external surfaces of nondisposable equipment in a dialysis unit, which of the following should be used?
   a. 1:100 bleach solution
   b. 1:100 vinegar solution
   c. 1:100 isopropyl alcohol solution
   d. 1:100 hydrochloric acid solution

10-5. Routine precautions for the care of the hemodialysis patient recommended by the CDC include:
   a. Patients should have specific dialysis stations assigned to them.
   b. Nondisposable items (such as chairs, etc.) must be cleaned at the end of each day.

    c. Medications should be prepared on a central medication cart and then taken to the patient's bedside.

    d. Clean and contaminated areas can be in the same area as long as they are clearly marked.

References

Case, C.L. (n.d.). Handwashing. *Access Excellence*. Retrieved August 16, 2010, from http://www.accessexcellence.org/AE/AEC/CC/hand_background.php

Centers for Disease Control and Prevention. (1998). Recommendations for prevention and control of hepatitis C virus (HCV) infections and HCV-related chronic disease. *MMWR, 47*(RR-19).

Centers for Disease Control and Prevention. (2001). Recommendations for preventing transmission of infections among chronic hemodialysis patients. *MMWR, 50*, 42.

Siegel, J.D., Rhinehart, E., Jackson, M., Chiarello, L., & the Healthcare Infection Control Practices Advisory Committee. (2007). Guideline for isolation precautions: Preventing transmission of infectious agents in healthcare settings. Retrieved from http://www.cdc.gov/ncidod/dhqp/pdf/isolation2007.pdf

Department of Health and Human Services, Centers for Medicare and Medicaid Services. (2008). Conditions for coverage for end-stage renal disease facilities: Final rule. *Federal Register*. Retrieved from www.cms.gov/CFCSAndCOPS/downloads/ESRDfinainile0415.pdf

New Jersey Administrative Code (N.J.A.C.). (n.d.). *Solid waste regulations*. 7:26–3A.6(b).

Medical Waste Disposal

11

This chapter includes topics on hazardous and medical waste. The methods of disposal of medical equipment and blood-saturated items are reviewed. There is discussion on the Williams-Steiger Occupational Safety and Health Act of 1970.

OBJECTIVES

1. Identify materials that constitute hazardous waste.
2. Identify materials that constitute medical waste.
3. Discuss methods of disposal for medical equipment.
4. Discuss methods of disposal for materials saturated with blood or body fluids.
5. Discuss sharps disposal.

PRE-TEST QUESTIONS

11-1. Wastes are considered hazardous if they are:
   a. Corrosive
   b. Malodorous
   c. Unsightly
   d. Liquids
11-2. Examples of medical wastes include all of the following *except*:
   a. Body parts removed during surgery
   b. Disposable, nonbloody patient gown
   c. Used hypodermic syringe
   d. Soiled wound dressing
11-3. Which of the following should be placed in a sharps container?
   a. Soiled wound dressing
   b. Empty vial that contained an injectable medication
   c. Syringe used to administer an intramuscular injection
   d. Used dialysis tubing

11-4. Medical wastes must be stored in a manner and location that protects the material from:
  a. Extreme cold temperatures
  b. Water
  c. Sunlight
  d. Earthquakes

11-5. Containers used for transporting medical waste should be:
  a. Flexible
  b. Designed to allow moisture to escape
  c. Porous
  d. Sealed

The Williams-Steiger Occupational Safety and Health Act of 1970 established the Occupational Safety and Health Administration (OSHA), which oversees federal standards for workplace safety. Subpart H of the OSHA standard deals specifically with hazardous materials. OSHA defines a *hazardous substance* as any material that, when exposed to, "results or may result in adverse affects on the health or safety of employees."

Wastes are listed as hazardous because they are known to be harmful to human health and the environment when not managed properly, regardless of their concentrations. Wastes may also be listed as hazardous it they exhibit certain characteristics, such as ignitability (creates a fire under certain conditions or is spontaneously combustible), corosivity (strong acids—pH less than or equal to 2, or strong bases—pH greater than or equal to 12.5), reactivity (unstable under normal conditions), or toxicity (harmful or fatal when ingested or absorbed). Congress delegated authority to regulate nuclear waste to the Nuclear Regulatory Commission (NRC) via the Atomic Energy Act of 1954. The safe handling and disposal of hazardous waste was given to the Environmental Protection Agency (EPA) in the Resource Conservation and Recovery Act of 1976 (RCRA). Some common examples of hazardous materials include mercury, cadmium, lead, strong acids and bases, combustible and flammable materials, oxygen, hydrogen, explosives, chlorinated organic compounds, as well as medical waste.

The Medical Waste Tracking Act of 1988, an amendment of the Solid Waste Disposal Act (MWTA) of the Environmental Protection Agency (EPA), defines *medical waste* as:

1. Cultures and stocks of infectious agents and associated biologicals, including cultures from medical and pathological laboratories, cultures and stock of infectious agents from research and industrial laboratories, wastes from the production of biologicals, discarded live and attenuated vaccines, and culture dishes and devises used to transfer, inoculate, and mix cultures (Figure 11.1).
2. Pathological wastes, including tissues, organs, and body parts that are removed during surgery or autopsy.
3. Waste human blood and products of blood, including serum, plasma, and other blood components (Figure 11.2).

FIGURE 11.1

Researcher handling infectious agents

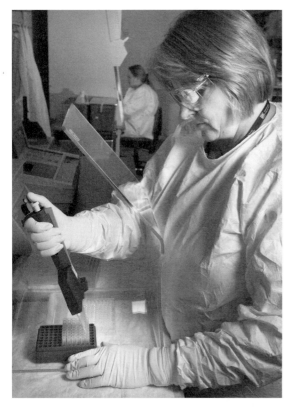

Courtesy of the Centers for Disease Control and Prevention / Hsi
Liu, PhD, MBA and James Gathany. Photo by James Gathany.

FIGURE 11.2

Syringe containing human amniotic fluid

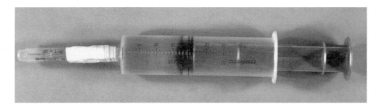

Courtesy of the Centers for Disease Control and Prevention / Dr. Andrew Chen.

4. Sharps that have been used in patient care or in medical, research, or industrial laboratories, including hypodermic needles, syringes, pastuer pi-
pettes, broken glass, and scalpel blades (Figure 11.3).

FIGURE 11.3

Phlebotomist disposing
of sharps materials after
performing a venipuncture
procedure

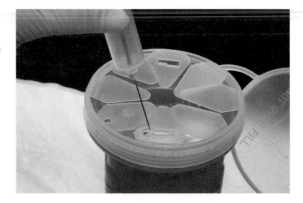

Courtesy of the Centers for Disease Control and Prevention. Photo by James Gathany.

5. Contaminated animal carcasses, body parts, and bedding of animals that were exposed to infectious agents during research, production of biologicals, or testing of pharmaceuticals.
6. Wastes from surgery or autopsy that were in contact with infectious agents, including soiled dressings, sponges, drapes, lavage tubes, drainage sets, underpads, and surgical gloves (Figure 11.4).
7. Laboratory waste from medical, pathological, pharmaceutical, or other research, commercial, or industrial laboratories that were in contact with infectious agents, including slides and covers slips, disposable gloves, laboratory coats, and aprons.
8. Dialysis wastes that were in contact with the blood of patients undergoing hemodialysis, including contaminated disposable equipment and supplies such tubing, filters, disposable sheets, towels gloves, aprons, and laboratory coats.
9. Discarded medical equipment and parts that were in contact with infectious agents.

FIGURE 11.4

Phlebotomist disposing of
gauze soiled with human
blood

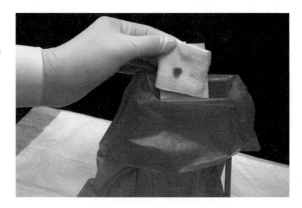

Courtesy of the Centers for Disease Control and Prevention. Photo by James Gathany.

10. Biological waste and discarded materials contaminated with blood, excretion, exudates, or secretion from human beings or animals that are isolated to protect others from communicable diseases.
11. Such other waste material that results from the administration of medical care to a patient by a health care provider and is found by the Administrator to posses a threat to human health or the environment.

CHARACTERISTICS OF HAZARDOUS WASTE

1. Ignitability: can produce fires under certain conditions, are spontaneously combustible, or have a flash point less than 140°F.
2. Corosivity: acids or bases that can dissolve metal containers.
3. Reactivity: unstable when heated, compressed, or mixed with water.
4. Toxicity: can produce illness or death when ingested or absorbed.

TYPES OF MEDICAL WASTE

1. Cultures and stocks from biologic and vaccine waste
2. Pathologic waste
3. Blood and blood products
4. Sharps
5. Contaminated animal products
6. Surgery and autopsy waste
7. Laboratory waste contaminated with infectious agents
8. Dialysis waste
9. Contaminated medical equipment
10. Other waste contaminated with infectious material

Most facilities that generate regulated medical waste transport these materials off-site for treatment and destruction. However, some facilities may process regulated medical waste on-site, thereby allowing them to dispose of these materials comingled with municipal solid waste.

All regulated medical waste must be segregated at the point of generation, typically into three categories: (a) sharps, including sharps containing residual fluid; (b) fluids; and (c) other solid waste. Sharps and nonsharps materials, such as fluids and solid regulated medical waste, may be included in sharps containers. These containers, even when mixed with nonsharps materials, are managed at all times as sharps containers. The waste in these containers should not be allowed to putrefy or become malodorous in any detectable manner. This is typically accomplished using refrigeration when necessary. If other nonregulated medical waste is placed in the same container(s) or cannot be segregated from regulated medical waste at the point of generation, then all the material must be packaged, labeled, and treated as regulated medical waste.

The containers used for transporting regulated medical waste must be rigid, leak-resistant, impervious to moisture, sufficiently strong to prevent tearing or breakage under normal conditions of use and handling, and sealed to prevent leakage during transport. Additionally, sharps and sharps with residual fluids must be placed in containers that are puncture resistant; and fluids must be packed in containers that completely seal and are break-resistant.

Medical waste must be stored in a manner and location that protects the materials and packaging from wind, water, and animals. The storage areas must be locked to prevent unauthorized access and must be maintained to prevent them from becoming breeding places or food sources for insects and rodents.

POST-TEST QUESTIONS

11-1. Wastes are considered hazardous if they are:
   a. Corrosive
   b. Malodorous
   c. Unsightly
   d. Liquids

11-2. Examples of medical wastes include all of the following *except*:
   a. Body parts removed during surgery
   b. Disposable, nonbloody patient gown
   c. Used hypodermic syringe
   d. Soiled wound dressing

11-3. Which of the following should be placed in a sharps container?
   a. Soiled wound dressing
   b. Empty vial that contained an injectable medication
   c. Syringe used to administer an intramuscular injection
   d. Used dialysis tubing

11-4. Medical wastes must be stored in a manner and location that protects the material from:
   a. Extreme cold temperatures
   b. Water
   c. Sunlight
   d. Earthquakes

11-5. Containers used for transporting medical waste should be:
   a. Flexible
   b. Designed to allow moisture to escape
   c. Porous
   d. Sealed

Reference

Report for H.R. 3515 Medical Waste Tracking Act of 1998. 100 Cong., 2 sess. January 25, 1988.

Web Site

http://www.cdc.gov/diabetes/pubs/images/laytest.gif

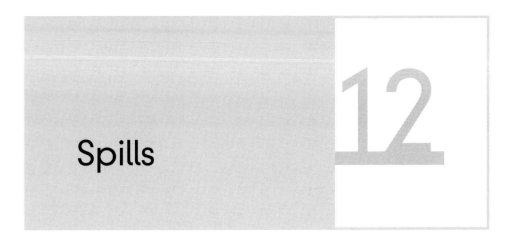

Spills

This chapter includes topics on the different types of spills in the health care setting. Blood spills and chemotherapy spills are reviewed. The content topics of the Hazard Communication Standard and the "right to know" law are reviewed. There is discussion on mercury spills.

OBJECTIVES

1. Create an action plan for a spill involving blood.
2. Create an action plan for a spill involving a chemotherapeutic agent.
3. Create an action plan for a spill involving mercury.
4. List three goals of the Hazard Communication Standard or "right to know" law.
5. List the information that can be found on a Material Data Safety Sheet.

PRE-TEST QUESTIONS

12-1. Which of the following agencies is responsible for overseeing hazardous exposures?
    a. Food and Drug Administration
    b. National Institutes of Health
    c. National Institute for Occupational Safety and Health
    d. Centers for Disease Control and Prevention
12-2. The blue area of National Fire Protection Association Rating system designates:
    a. Health risks
    b. Flammability risks
    c. Instability risks
    d. Which personal protective equipment (PPE) is needed
12-3. Which of the following categories of information is provided on a Material Data Safety Sheet?
    a. Spill procedure
    b. Health hazard data

     c. Flammability information

     d. All of the above

12-4. Which of the following is necessary to clean a blood spill?

     a. Sodium hypochlorite

     b. Sulfur

     c. Vinegar

     d. Acetone

12-5. Which of the following is necessary to clean a mercury spill?

     a. Sodium hypochlorite

     b. Sulfur

     c. Vinegar

     d. Acetone

A *spill* is defined as a hazard that results from a contamination of harmful or potentially harmful substances. In the United States, two organizations oversee hazardous exposures—the National Institute for Occupational Safety and Health (NIOSH) and the Occupational Safety and Health Administration (OSHA). In 1974, NIOSH joined OSHA in developing a series of occupational health standards for substances with existing permissible exposure limits (PELs). NIOSH is responsible for recommending health and safety standards, while OSHA is responsible for dissemination and enforcement actions. NIOSH also makes recommendations to prevent, reduce, and/or eliminate the adverse health effects of workplace chemical and accidental injuries. (For the most current information and updates, consult the electronic version on the NIOSH Web site: http://www.cdc.gov/niosh/npg/npg.html)

Toxic exposures can involve solid, liquid, or gaseous hazardous materials. Although the discussion of exposure and exposure limits that follows in the next two paragraphs is most easily understood when considering airborne contaminations, these concepts apply to solid and liquid materials, as well. Airborne concentrations are given in parts per million (ppm), milligrams per cubic meter (mg/m3) and millions of particles per cubic foot of air (mppcf).

NIOSH acts under the authority of the Occupational Safety and Health Act of 1970 (29USC Chapter 15) and the Federal Mine Safety and Health Act of 1977 (30 USC Chapter 22) and develops and periodically revises recommended exposure limits (RELs) for hazardous substances or conditions in the workplace. For NIOSH RELs, a time-weighted average (TWA) concentration for up to a 10-hour workday during a 40-hour work week is also designated, as well as a short-term exposure limit (STEL). The STEL is a 15-minute TWA exposure that should not be exceeded at any time during a workday. A ceiling REL should not be exceeded at any time. TWA concentrations for OSHA PELs must not be exceeded during any 8-hour workshift of a 40-hour work week. In addition, there are a number of substances that have PEL ceiling values that must not be exceeded except for specified excursions. For example, a "5-minute maximum peak in any 2 hours" means that a 5-minute exposure above the ceiling value, but never above the maximum peak, is allowed in any 2 hours during an 8-hour workday.

Substances that pose an immediate danger to life or health (IDLH) are given special attention. NIOSH has established IDLH criteria, which are meant to determine the airborne concentration from which a worker could escape without injury or irreversible health effects from an IDLH exposure in the event of respiratory protective equipment failure. These injuries include reversible effects, such as severe eye or respiratory irritation, and disorientation, which might prevent escape. The IDLH values are based on the consequences of a 30-minute exposure. **Be advised**—the 30-minute period was instituted as a safety margin and is *not* meant to imply that it is safe for workers to remain in the hazardous environment for that time period. ***Every effort should be made to exit immediately!***

In addition to standard work place practices, such as no eating, drinking, chewing gum, smoking, applying make-up, or other personal grooming, NIOSH designates the additional types of personal protective equipment (PPE) that should be used when handling or exposed to a potentially hazardous substance. These include the need for personal protective clothing and the need for eye protection. Additionally, NIOSH also indicates additional protective measures to be taken, such as recommending when workers should wash the spilled chemical from the body in addition to normal washing (e.g., before eating), advising workers when to remove clothing that has accidentally become wet or significantly contaminated, whether routine changing of clothing is needed, or when eyewash fountains and/or quick drench facilities are needed.

All spills are handled in essentially the same manner. Make sure that you notify the appropriate personnel at your facility of the spill to prevent additional accidental exposure, and protect yourself by donning the appropriate PPE for the spill. Remember that risk is minimized when you are wearing the proper PPE for the potential exposure, such as gloves, gown, and/or face/eye shield (Figure 12.1).

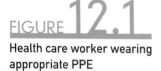

FIGURE 12.1

Health care worker wearing appropriate PPE

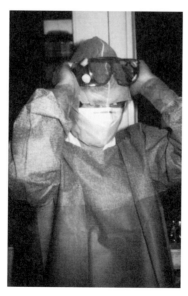

Courtesy of the Centers for Disease Control and Prevention / Dr. J. Lyle Conrad.

HANDLING SPILLS

1. Notify coworkers of the spill.
2. Don PPE.
3. Contain the spill.
4. Clean the spill.
5. Dispose of the spill.

BLOOD SPILLS

Small blood spills can easily be managed by covering with a disposable cleaning rag saturated with a 1:100 (500 ppm) sodium hypochlorite solution. Allow this to sit while you don appropriate PPE, then wipe the spill, and dispose of the rag. Larger blood spills should be cleaned with a mop and disinfection-grade cleaning solution. Remember, the mop head needs to be replaced or sanitized before used in other areas.

CHEMOTHERAPEUTIC AGENTS

The risk to individuals working with hazardous drugs is a function of the extent of exposure and the toxicity profile of the hazardous drug. While pharmacies and their staff typically mix and prepare chemotherapy, it is not uncommon to have other health care workers (HCW) involved in this process, especially in smaller institutions and outpatient settings. Injectable drugs can splatter or become airborne during any of the usual processes of drug administration, such as needle withdrawal from the medication vial, expulsion of air from the drug-filled syringe, or transfer of the drug from the needle syringe to the intravenous infusion bag. If the medication is delivered in an ampule, the process of breaking open the ampule can be a source of contamination. Oral chemotherapy can also pose a risk to HCW and should never be handled, with or without gloves. Gloves will not necessarily protect you because all glove materials are permeable to some hazardous drugs. Accidental ingestion by the worker can occur when his or her food and/or cigarettes becomes contaminated.

Contaminated materials used in the preparation and administration of these drugs, such as gloves, gowns, syringes, needles, and vials, pose a risk to support staff and housekeeping services. Disposal of some of these agents is regulated by the EPA (see Chapter 11, "Medical Waste Disposal").

Patients receiving chemotherapeutic agents excrete these potentially hazardous materials in their secretions (urine, feces, others). As such, personnel handle linens and clothing that may be contaminated. These individuals must protect themselves by wearing double latex gloves (found to be the least permeable of glove material) and disposable, waterproof gowns. Eye protection should be worn if splashing is possible. Hands must be washed after glove removal and after contact with these substances. Linen and clothing should be placed into designated laundry bags and the laundry bags placed into an impervious bag for transport. The laundry bag and its contents should be prewashed, and then the linens and clothing can be added to other laundry for a second wash.

Hazardous drug spills are divided into small and large spills using the 5 mL or 5 gm size as the cutoff. Spills with volumes less than 5 mL are considered small, while those containing more than 5 mL of contaminated material are considered large. Spill kits should be readily available to manage these events. Spills must be cleaned immediately by personnel wearing gowns, double latex gloves, and splash goggles. If airborne substances may be generated, a NIOSH-approved respirator should be used. Small spills should be wiped up with an absorbent gauze pad. The spill area should then be cleaned three times using a detergent solution followed by clean water. Large spills should be contained by gently covering the spill with disposable absorbent sheets or pillows. If a dry spill has occurred, disposable damp cloths or towels should be used. Remember to be gentle in your application and cleaning procedure to prevent additional splashing or aerosolization of the spill material.

Chemotherapy Spill Kit Contents

1. Chemical splash goggles
2. Two pairs of latex gloves
3. Utility gloves
4. Low-permeability gown
5. Two sheets (12" x 12") of absorbent material
6. 250-mL and 1-liter spill control pillows
7. Sharps container
8. Small scoop to collect glass fragments
9. Two large waste disposal bags

MERCURY

Mercury can be found in a variety of commercial and household items, such as blood pressure monitors, thermometers, thermostats, and fluorescent light bulbs. The mercury content of these items (see Table 12.1) varies from as little as a few milligrams (fluorescent light bulbs) to as much as hundreds of grams (sphygmomanometers). When liquid elemental mercury is spilled, it forms beads that travel and accumulate in cracks and other tiny places. The spilled mercury also vaporizes, posing both a hazard to skin as well as a respiratory hazard. Most small mercury spills (less than 30 mL of mercury) can be easily cleaned. Large spills need to be cleaned by an industrial professional. *Never use a household vacuum or shop vacuum to clean up a mercury spill.* The vacuum disseminates mercury vapors, increasing the exposure risk. Contaminated vacuums need to be taken to a mercury collection program.

As with other spills, notify others, contain the spill, and use a spill kit if available. Keep the room below 70 degrees F to minimize mercury evaporation. Contain the spill using disposable rags. Prevent the mercury from moving into drains,

TABLE **12.1**

Mercury Content of Selected Items

ITEM	MERCURY CONTENT
Fever Thermometers	0.5 gm
Laboratory Thermometers	3 gms
Thermostats	3 gms
Tilt Switches	3–4 gms
Float Switches	2 gms
Fluorescent Light Bulbs	5–250 mg
Button Batteries	25 mg

cracks, or onto sloped or porous surfaces. If glass is involved, use tweezers to pick up broken glass and place it into secure container. Do not use a broom to sweep up the mercury as it will break up the mercury into smaller pieces. Work from the outside of the spill area toward the center gently pushing the mercury to form larger beads. Push the mercury into a plastic dustpan. Shine a flashlight to look for additional glass or mercury beads, which will reflect the light. Once the mercury is cleaned up, apply sulfur powder to the spill area. If mercury is still present, there will be a color change from bright yellow to brown, indicating more clean-up is needed. Dispose of all contaminated items into a wide-mouthed plastic container with a screw-top lid. Ventilate the room to the outside air to eliminate residual mercury vapors.

Mercury Spill Kit Contents

1. Latex gloves
2. Tweezers
3. Goggles
4. Disposable rags
5. Rubber squeegee
6. Plastic dust pan
7. Wide-mouth plastic container with screw-top lid
8. Flashlight
9. Eye dropper or other suction device
10. Sulfur powder

HAZARDOUS COMMUNICATION

In 1994 OSHA finalized the Hazard Communication Standard (29 CFR 1920.1200), otherwise known as the "right to know" law. This standard requires employers to establish a hazard communication programs informing employees of the hazards and identities of the chemicals that they may be exposed to in the workplace. These communication programs also include the protective measures that workers can take to protect themselves from chemical adverse effects. The goals of the hazard communication are to reduce the risks in working with hazardous materials, improve the communication of vital information about these hazards, reduce illnesses and injuries associated with hazardous materials, and reduce the volume and toxicity of hazardous material exposure.

Chemical hazards are classified as physical hazards, health hazards, or both. Chemicals that pose physical hazards include those that can result in fire or explosion. Health hazards can be classified as *acute hazards,* producing effects after short-term exposure such as burns or poisonings, or chronic hazards, which occur after long-term exposure and include cancer and heart disease as examples. Some commonly encountered chemical hazards that HCWs are exposed to include anesthetic agents, ethylene oxide (a sterilant used for medical supplies and equipment), oxygen, mercury, formaldehyde, glutaraldehyde (a disinfectant used to decontaminate medical equipment), and anticancer drugs.

Physical Hazards That Produce Fire or Explosion

- Combustible liquids
- Compressed gas
- Explosive agents
- Flammable substances
- Organic peroxides
- Oxidizers
- Pyrophoric agents
- Unstable compounds
- Water-reactive substances

Health Hazards

- Carcinogens
- Toxic or highly toxic agents
- Reproductive toxins
- Irritants
- Corrosives
- Sensitizers
- Nephrotoxins
- Neurotoxins
- Agents that act on the hematopoietic system
- Agents that may damage lungs, skin, eyes, or mucus membranes

Every employer must ensure that a Material Data Safety Sheet (MSDS) is present for every product that is used in the workplace (see Figure 12.2). The

FIGURE **12.2**
Material Data Safety Sheet

Material Safety Data Sheet

I Product:	BLEACH
Description:	CLEAR ALKALINE LIQUID WITH A CHLORINE ODOR

Other Designations	Distributor	Emergency Telephone Nos.
Sodium Hypochlorite Bleach		

II Health Hazard Data

CORROSIVE to the eyes. Injures eyes, skin and mucous membranes on contact. Harmful if swallowed; nausea, vomiting, and burning sensation of the mouth and throat may occur. No adverse health effects are expected with recommended use. Occasional clinical reports suggest a low potential for sensitization upon exaggerated exposure to sodium hypochlorite if skin damage (e.g. irritation) occurs during exposure. However, clinical tests conducted on intact skin using a product similar found no sensitization in the test subjects.

Although not expected, heart conditions or chronic respiratory problems such as asthma, chronic bronchitis or obstructive lung disease may be aggravated by exposure to high concentrations of vapor or mist.

FIRST AID:

EYE CONTACT: Immediately flush eyes with water for 15 minutes. If irritation persists, call a doctor.

SKIN CONTACT: Remove contaminated clothing. Flush skin with water. If irritation persists, call a doctor.

INGESTION: Drink a glassful of water. DO NOT induce vomiting. Immediately contact a doctor or poison control center.

INHALATION: Remove from exposure to fresh air. If breathing problems develop, call a doctor.

III Hazardous Ingredients

Ingredient	Concentration	Worker Exposure Limit
Sodium hypochlorite CAS # 7681-52-9	5-10%	not established
Sodium hydroxide CAS # 1310-73-2	0.1-1%	2 mg/m^3 - TLV-C^a 2 mg/m^3 - PEL-TWA^b

^{a}TLV-C = ACGIH Threshold Limit Value - Ceiling

^{b}PEL-TWA = OSHA Permissible Exposure Limit - Time Weighted Average/Short Term Exposure Limit

None of the ingredients in this product are on the IARC, OSHA or NTP carcinogen lists.

IV Special Protection and Precautions

Hygienic Practices: Wash hands after direct contact. Do not wear product-contaminated clothing for prolonged periods.

Engineering Controls: Use local exhaust to minimize exposure to product vapor or mist.

Personal Protective Equipment: Wear safety glasses. Wear rubber or neoprene gloves if there is the potential for repeated or prolonged skin contact. In situations where exposure limits may be exceeded, a NIOSH-approved respirator is advised.

V Transportation and Regulatory Data

DOT: Not restricted per 49 CFR 172.101(c)(12)(iv).

IMDG: Not restricted per IMDG Code Page 0021 Paragraph 5.3.5.

IATA: Not restricted per IATA D.G.R. Special Provision A3.

EPA - SARA TITLE III/CERCLA: This product is regulated under Sections 311/312 and contains no chemicals reportable under Section 313. This product does contain chemicals (sodium hydroxide and sodium hypochlorite) that are regulated under Section 304/CERCLA.

TSCA/DSL STATUS: All components of this product are on the U.S. TSCA Inventory and Canadian DSL.

VI Spill Procedures/Waste Disposal

Spill Procedures: Absorb and containerize. Wash residual down to sanitary sewer. Contact the sanitary treatment facility in advance to assure ability to process washed-down material. For spills of multiple products, responders should evaluate the MSDS's of the products for incompatibility with sodium hypochlorite. Breathing protection should be worn in enclosed, and/or poorly ventilated areas until hazard assessment is complete.

Waste Disposal: Dispose must be made in accordance with applicable federal, state and local regulations.

VII Reactivity Data

Stable under normal use and storage conditions. Reacts with other household chemicals such as toilet bowl cleaners, rust removers, acids or ammonia containing products to produce hazardous gases, such as chlorine and other chlorinated species. Prolonged contact with metals may cause pitting or discoloration.

VIII Fire and Explosion Data

Not flammable or explosive.

IX Physical Data

pH...

Specific gravity (H$_2$0=1) ....

Solubility in water ....

DATA SUPPLIED IS FOR USE ONLY IN CONNECTION WITH OCCUPATIONAL SAFETY AND HEALTH

MSDS lists the product's chemical components, it's dangers, and how to work safely with it. The MSDS is provided by the manufacturer and must be sent with the first product shipment and anytime the information about the product changes. OSHA does not mandate the order or the format of the MSDS, only its content. The heading area provides the chemical name, date of issue of the MSDS, and the name, address, and telephone number of the manufacturer. The material identification section gives the generic names of the product and the National Fire Protection Association (NFPA) hazardous rating (see Figure 12.3), which provides flammability, reactivity, and health hazard information for fire fighters and emergency response agencies displayed in a diamond divided into four colored sections. This should be differentiated from the Hazardous Material Identification System (HMIS), which uses a square-shaped icon composed of four colored bars (see Figure 12.4).

The hazard section of the MSDS names each dangerous substance, the concentration percentage, and the safe exposure limits, that is, PEL for an 8-hour workday, STEL for a 15-minute average exposure, and the ceiling limit, which should never be exceeded. The physical data section identifies the product as a solid, liquid, or gas and gives its physical appearance and physical properties, such as the freezing point, melting point, boiling point, vapor pressure, and evaporation rate. The fire and explosion data include the flash point, flammability (if the product can ignite at temperatures below 100°F), and combustibility (if the product can catch fire above 100°F). Reactivity data provides information about what happens if the product contacts air, water, or other agents and if there are incompatibilities with these agents. The health hazard section provides information about the route of entry, symptoms of overexposure, if an over-exposure worsens existing medical conditions, the acute and chronic health effects, if the product is carcinogenic, and the medical and first aid treatments. Spill, leak, and disposal procedures describe the containment methods, clean-up procedures, and emergency equipment needed. Special protection includes the methods to reduce exposure, ventilation requirements, protective clothing, and instructions for care and disposal of contaminated equipment.

Content of MSDS

- Chemical identity
- Material identification
- Hazards
- Physical data
- Fire and explosive data
- Reactivity data
- Health hazards
- Spill, leak and disposal procedures
- Special protection information
- Special precautions and comments
- Storage and handling procedures

FIGURE **12.3**

National Fire Protection Association Rating

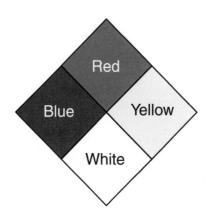

Health Hazard (Blue Area): Rated 0 to 4

4 - Very short exposure could cause death or serious residual injury even though prompt medical attention was given.

3 - Short exposure could cause serious temporary or residual injury even though prompt medical attention was given.

2 - Intense or continued exposure could cause temporary incapacitation or possible residual injury unless prompt medical attention is given.

1 - Exposure could cause irritation but only minor residual injury even if no treatment is given.

0 - Exposure under fire conditions would offer no hazard beyond that of ordinary combustible materials.

Flammability (Red Area): Rated 0 to 4

4 - Will rapidly or completely vaporize at normal pressure and temperature, or is readily dispersed in air and will burn readily.

3 - Liquids and solids that can be ignited under almost all ambient conditions.

2 - Must be moderately heated or exposed to relatively high temperature before ignition can occur.

1 - Must be preheated before ignition can occur.

0 - Materials that will not burn.

(continued)

FIGURE **12.3**

(*Continued*)

Instability (Yellow Area): Rated 0 to 4

4 - Readily capable of detonation or of explosive decomposition or reaction at normal temperatures and pressures.
3 - Capable of detonation or explosive reaction, but requires a strong initiating source or must be heated under confinement before initiation, or reacts explosively with water.
2 - Normally unstable and readily undergo violent decomposition but do not detonate. Also: may react violently with water or may form potentially explosive mixtures with water.
1 - Normally stable, but can become unstable at elevated temperatures and pressures or may react with water with some release of energy, but not violently.
0 - Normally stable, even under fire exposure conditions, and are not reactive with water.

Special Hazards (White Area)

OX – This denotes an oxidizer, a chemical that can greatly increase the rate of combustion or fire.
SA - This denotes gases that are simple asphyxiants. The only gases for which this symbol is permitted are nitrogen, helium, neon, argon, krypton, and xenon. The use of this hazard symbol is optional.
W - This denotes unusual reactivity with water. This indicates a potential hazard using water to fight a fire involving this material. When a compound is both water-reactive and an oxidizer, the W symbol should go in this quadrant and the OX warning is placed immediately below the NFPA diamond.

FIGURE 12.4

Hazardous Material Identification System

Health	☐ ☐
Flammability	☐
Reactivity	
Personal Protection	

Blue Area:
  An * in the first box indicates chronic health hazard
  Rated 0 (minimum) to 4 (severe) in the second box

Red Area:
  Rated 0 (minimum) to 4 (severe)

Yellow Area:
  Rated 0 (minimum) to 4 (severe)

White Area:
  Coded A to Z for type of required personal protection

POST-TEST QUESTIONS

12-1. Which of the following agencies is responsible for overseeing hazardous exposures?
  a. Food and Drug Administration
  b. National Institutes of Health
  c. National Institute for Occupational Safety and Health
  d. Centers for Disease Control and Prevention

12-2. The blue area of National Fire Protection Association Rating system designates:
  a. Health risks
  b. Flammability risks
  c. Instability risks
  d. Which PPE is needed

12-3. Which of the following categories of information is provided on a Material Data Safety Sheet?
  a. Spill procedure
  b. Health hazard data
  c. Flammability information
  d. All of the above

12-4. Which of the following is necessary to clean a blood spill?
  a. Sodium hypochlorite
  b. Sulfur
  c. Vinegar
  d. Acetone

12-5. Which of the following is necessary to clean a mercury spill?
  a. Sodium hypochlorite
  b. Sulfur
  c. Vinegar
  d. Acetone

Web Site

http://www.cdc.gov/niosh/npg/npg.html

13

Methods of Surveillance

This chapter includes topics on active and passive infectious disease surveillance and the tracking of multidrug-resistant organisms. Examples of surveillance efforts and vaccine safety are reviewed. The content differentiates between a cohort study and a case control study. There is discussion on the performance improvement process and how it relates to methods of surveillance. Finally, sentinel, vector, risk factor surveillance, and improved outcomes with early detection are discussed.

OBJECTIVES

1. List the benefits of infectious disease surveillance.
2. Explain how to calculate the mean, median, and mode for a given data set.
3. Describe the difference between a cohort study and a case control study.
4. Explain how to fill a two-by-two table and calculate sensitivity, specificity, positive predictive value, and negative predictive value.
5. List the members of a typical surveillance team and their roles.
6. Name the steps in the performance improvement process.

PRE-TEST QUESTIONS

13-1. Which of the following types of surveillance relies on data collected from a subset of the population that can then be generalized back to the broader population?
a. Administrative surveillance
b. Vector surveillance
c. Laboratory-based surveillance
d. Sentinel surveillance

13-2. What is calculated by adding the list of values and dividing by the number of values in the data set?
a. Mean
b. Median

   c. Mode

   d. Benchmark

13-3. What study type identifies all cases by "looking backward" using a chart review?

   a. Longitudinal

   b. Cross-sectional

   c. Prospective

   d. Retrospective

13-4. Which of the following refers to the proportion of patients with the disease who have a positive test result?

   a. Specificity

   b. Sensitivity

   c. Positive predictive value

   d. Negative predictive value

13-5. What does the "D" stand for in the PDCA cycle?

   a. Debate

   b. Discover

   c. Do

   d. Deliver

Surveillance is the cornerstone to all infection prevention and control activities. Surveillance assists in highlighting areas of concern relative to the identification, transmission, and control of infectious agents, as well as processes that can be improved and tracking progress after improvement programs have been instituted (Table 13.1). Surveillance can be local, such as those performed in a doctor's office or a specific ward in a long-term care facility; or it can be more broadly based on a community, state, national, or global level.

There are many types of surveillance efforts (M'ikanatha et al., 2007). Surveillance can either be active or passive. *Active* surveillance is initiated and

TABLE **13.1**

Examples of Surveillance Efforts

- Determination of the strains of seasonal influenza for vaccine preparation
- Vaccination strategies
- Vaccine safety
- Track multidrug-resistant organisms (MDROs)
- Limit the spread of MDROs
- Identify and track infectious outbreaks, such as the H1N1 pandemic

driven by public health efforts to identify and track cases. These surveys usually capture 100% of the data. *Passive* surveillance, on the other hand, is provider initiated and usually has limited involvement of the public health system. Although passive surveillance may be designed to capture the entire data set, these efforts are usually more limited in scope. *Sentinel* surveillance relies on data collected from a subset of the population. This type of population sampling limits the resources necessary for data collection without limiting the ability to generalize the data back to the broader population. An example might be the use of a single Medical / Surgical ward in a hospital as a sentinel site to track and analyze the number of health care–associated infections (HAI) in order to determine if there is a problem in the hospital as a whole. *Vector* surveillance examines the role of insects in the spread of infectious disease. Similarly, *animal* surveillance examines the roles of animals and other wildlife in disease transmission. *Risk factor* surveillance focuses on the genetic, environmental, and behavioral risks for disease acquisition, for example, sexual activity patterns in women and their risk for cervical cancer. *Laboratory-based* surveillance and *administrative* surveillance utilize preexisting data, such as antibiotic sensitivity from cultures processed by the microbiological laboratory or the patterns of antibiotic use among members of a health maintenance organization (HMO).

Data that are collected and analyzed need to be discreet and measurable—reducing the chances of interobserver and intraobserver variability. Similarly, case definitions must not be vague.

Case Study 1

Dr. Wellbee, a successful pediatrician, noticed that the boys he was seeing were taller than the girls. He decided to perform a surveillance activity. He added a check box to the top of his intake form that read "Tall: ◆ YES ◆ NO". His nurses, Mary, Susan, and John began indicating whether each child that they cared for was "tall" or not. The system was working well until Dr. Wellbee began to analyze the data and saw Sam Hill's name appear twice. Sam had a runny nose and his mother brought him in for a check-up and follow-up visit. Mary did the first intake and noted that Sam was "tall"; John did the intake for the follow-up visit and checked the "no" box, meaning Sam was not tall.

A better case definition might have utilized the pediatric growth chart and defined a tall child as one who was above the 90th percentile for height. Such a definition eliminates the subjective bias of the observer (in this case the nurse performing the intake) and improves the reliability of the data.

MEASURES OF CENTRAL TENDENCY

The information contained in a data set can be communicated in a variety of ways. For a working group the raw data are often reviewed and analyzed for patterns and trends. This allows the individual members to form their own opinions about the data. When the data set is very large, this type of review is often cumbersome and difficult. Instead, we use other measures of central tendency to convey information about the set as a whole without having to look at all the individual values. The three most commonly used measures of central tendency are the mean, median, and mode.

Case Study 2: Reporting the Average Using the Mean Value

Dr. Wellbee met with his nurses, John, Mary, and Susan. They refined their surveillance activity by tracking the actual height of their patients. They decided to collect and review the heights of all children each day. Mary prepares Table 13.2, listing all patients' first names, whether they are boys or girls, and their heights. She also reports that the average or mean height of all the children seen on Monday, March 1, was 35.5 inches; for the girls, 31.7 inches; and for the boys, 39.8 inches. The mean is calculated by summing or adding the list of values and dividing by the number of values in the data set.

TABLE **13.2**

First Name, Sex and Height of All Patients Seen on March 1

MONDAY MARCH 1		
NAME	SEX	HEIGHT
Sam	Boy	45"
Jill	Girl	32"
Brian	Boy	40"
Tom	Boy	38"
Wendy	Girl	12"
Susan	Girl	38"
Sarah	Girl	32"
Bob	Boy	36"
Todd	Boy	42"
Jack	Boy	38"
Mary	Girl	38"
Alice	Girl	36"
Betty	Girl	34"

Case Study 3: Reporting the Average Using the Median Value

John is surprised. He listed the heights in order for the boys, 36, 38, 38, 40, 42, 45, and guessed that the average height would be about 39 inches; and for the girls, 12, 32, 32, 34, 36, 38, 38, and guessed that their average height would be about 34 inches. Why did Mary have an average height for the girls that differed so much from John's? Dr. Wellbee explained that Mary reported the average by calculating the mean value while John calculated the median.

The median is calculated by first placing the list of values into rank order and then choosing the middle value if there is an odd number of values (such as the list for girls' heights); or, if there is an even number of values (such as the list for boys' heights), summing the two middle values and dividing by 2. Another method of describing sets of values uses the mode. The mode indicates the value or values that occur most often in a data set. In this example, the mode would be 38 for the boys and 32 and 38 for girls. If the data set is represented graphically, the mode gives you an idea about the shape of the curve.

Case Study 4: Describing the Data Using the Mode

Dr. Wellbee asked Susan, John, and Mary to help him with another project. He suspects that his teenage patients are not being vaccinated for seasonal influenza. They agree to collect and review the data of all children seen on Friday, April 2. There will be three doctors working that day, and each nurse will be assigned to a different doctor. John puts all of the data into Table 13.3, listing the nurse who cared for the patient at the visit, patient age, and seasonal influenza vaccination status ranked by patient age. John decides to list all infants as age 0 for simplicity.

TABLE 13.3

Distribution of Nurse Providing Patient Care, Patient Age and Vaccination Status

NURSE	PATIENT AGE	VACCINE STATUS
John	0	Y
John	1	Y
Mary	1	Y

(Continued)

TABLE 13.3

(*Continued*)

NURSE	PATIENT AGE	VACCINE STATUS
Susan	2	Y
John	2	Y
John	2	Y
Mary	3	Y
Susan	3	Y
Mary	3	Y
John	3	Y
Mary	4	Y
John	4	Y
Susan	4	Y
John	5	Y
John	5	Y
John	5	Y
Mary	6	N
Susan	7	Y
Susan	7	Y
John	7	Y
Mary	9	N
Mary	9	N
Susan	9	Y
Susan	9	Y
John	11	Y
Susan	11	Y
John	13	N
Mary	13	N
Mary	13	N
Mary	14	N

(*Continued*)

TABLE 13.3
(Continued)

NURSE	PATIENT AGE	VACCINE STATUS
Mary	14	N
Susan	14	N
Susan	14	N
John	15	Y
Mary	15	N
Mary	15	N
Susan	15	Y
Susan	16	Y
Susan	17	Y
Mary	18	N
Susan	18	N
John	19	N

DATA DISTRIBUTION AND SKEWNESS

When the mean, median, and mode are all the same value, the data set is described as being normally distributed. A normal distribution is often called a Gaussian distribution by physicists because Gauss used this distribution in his studies of astronomical data in 1809 (Weisstein, n.d.). Given its shape, social scientists refer to this distribution as a bell curve. A normal distribution is symmetric around the mean, median, and mode.

Dr. Wellbee asks John to create a histogram of all the patient ages so that he can see the distribution of the ages (see Figure 13.1). Dr. Wellbee also asks for a similar histogram for those patients who have not been vaccinated as well as for those who have (see Figures 13.2 and 13.3).

Dr. Wellbee comments that the histogram for those patients who have not been vaccinated for seasonal influenza is normally distributed (see Figure 13.4). He shows his staff the corresponding data table to make his point. He shows them that the median and mode age are both 14. He then demonstrates that the mean age is also 14 by summing all the ages (6 + 9 + 9 + 13 + 13 + 13, etc.), which equals 216, and then dividing 216 by the total number of patients (16), arriving at the result 13.5, which rounds up to 14 (see Table 13.4).

FIGURE 13.1

Distribution of patient age for visits on April 2

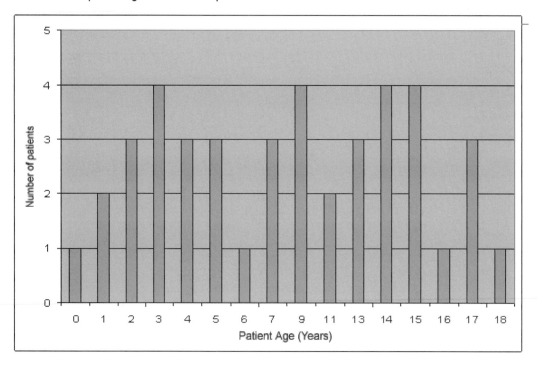

FIGURE 13.2

Distribution of patient age for patients not vaccinated for seasonal influenza on April 2

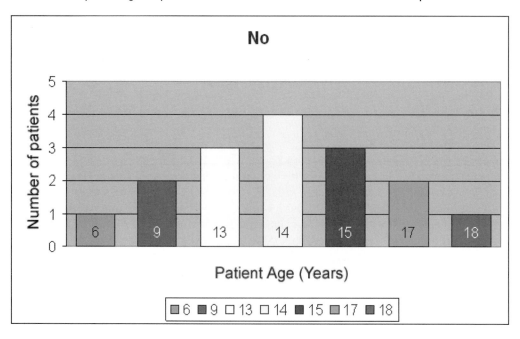

FIGURE 13.3

Distribution of patient age for patients vaccinated for seasonal influenza on April 2

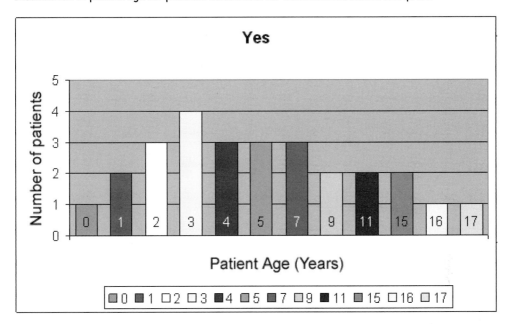

FIGURE 13.4

Normal distribution

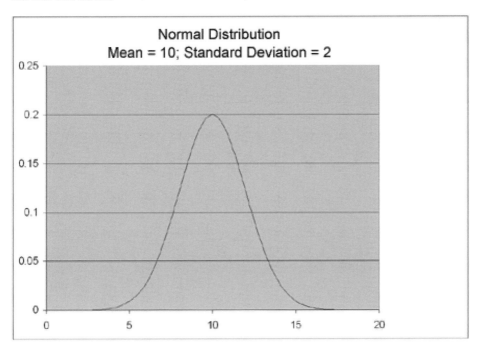

TABLE **13.4**

Number of Patients in Each Age Category Who Were Not Vaccinated for Seasonal Influenza and Who Presented for an Office Visit on April 2

PATIENT AGE	COUNT
6	1
9	2
13	3
14	4
15	3
17	2
18	1

He then explains that the histogram for the patients who were vaccinated for seasonal influenza is not normally distributed but is positively skewed. Data that are positively skewed have values that are clustered to the left of center. The mean values fall to the right of the median and give the highest estimate of central tendency, and the mode values fall to the left of the median and give the

TABLE **13.5**

Number of Patients in Each Age Category Who Were Vaccinated for Seasonal Influenza and Who Presented for an Office Visit on April 2

PATIENT AGE	COUNT
0	1
1	2
2	3
3	4
4	3
5	3
7	3
9	2
11	2
15	2
16	1
17	1

lowest estimate of central tendency. Negatively skewed data have the opposite characteristics. Once again, Dr. Wellbee utilizes the corresponding data table (see Table 13.5). He shows them that the mode age is 3. He then demonstrates that the mean age is 7 by once again summing all the ages (0 + 1 + 1 + 2 + 2 + 2, etc.), which equals 171, and then dividing this by the total number of patients (27), resulting in a mean age of 6.3, which rounds down to 6. Dr. Wellbee points out for those who are interested that the median age happens to be 5.

TYPES OF SURVEILLANCE

There are a variety of ways to collect surveillance data (see Table 13.6). Each of the different methods has varying time requirements and offers certain advantages that will allow you to draw certain conclusions from the data set. The types of surveys that can be performed include longitudinal surveys, cross-sectional studies, prospective studies, and retrospective studies (Gastmeier, Coignard, & Horan, 2007).

A longitudinal survey usually captures a complete data set for the period in question. It allows you to calculate incidence rates and assists in the identification of risk factors. This type of surveillance is extremely time consuming and labor intensive.

A cross-sectional study captures the prevalence rates for the disease in question. It provides you with a "snap-shot" look at the population in question. It is usually performed as a "first-look" because it is not as time consuming or labor intensive as a longitudinal survey. The data derived from a cross-sectional study can be compared with a published benchmark. If a problem is identified in your population, a more detailed data collection can then be performed.

A prospective survey identifies all cases (meeting the case definition) "looking forward" from a given point in time. This type of survey allows for a complete

TABLE **13.6**

Types of Surveillance Studies

SURVEILLANCE TYPE	TIME REQUIREMENT	ABILITY TO PROVE CAUSALITY
Longitudinal Survey	++++	++++
Prospective Study	++++	+++
Cohort Study	+++	++
Retrospective Study	++	+
Case-Control Study	++	+
Cross-sectional Survey	+	+

collection of data and, like the longitudinal survey, is both time consuming and labor intensive.

A cohort study looks at a group of patients who have one or more common features. These features may be demographic in nature (white females, or men over the age of 50); they may represent a shared clinical event (patients with hemoglobin below 10 gm/dL, or patients on hemodialysis) or a common administrative detail.

A retrospective survey identifies all cases "looking backward" within a specified time period. It is usually performed as a chart review or the review of administrative or laboratory data. Retrospective surveys take less time than prospective surveys and are limited by the data that exists within the established record. If key data elements are not completely recorded, the validity of the conclusion drawn is called into question.

A case-control study is a retrospective, observational study that looks at patients with a similar condition (case) and compares them to similarly matched patients who do not have the condition (controls) to determine the relationship between exposure to a particular risk factor and the development of a certain condition. While this type of surveillance effort does not require a significant amount of time, it does not allow you to prove a cause-and-effect relationship.

How Do You Do It

Initiating a surveillance effort may, at the outset, seem like a daunting task. However, a few basic steps will help keep you organized and simplify the process. First and foremost, establish your team. The surveillance team is typically headed by the infection control and prevention (ICP) professional. Other team members may include individuals from the laboratory, clinicians such as doctors and nurses, the local administrators as well as the local public health department. Each member of the team should have a defined role and responsibility. The second item to address is the identification of the disease or problem to be studied. The team generally identifies the areas of concern or those that may need review. These are usually conditions that have one or more of the following characteristics: they pose a high risk for morbidity or mortality, they are present in high numbers in your population, options are available for disease prevention and/or treatment, and early detection and treatment is associated with improved outcomes. The team may choose to collect baseline data and compare values against local or national benchmarks to identify areas for study.

Choosing a Disease for Surveillance

High risk of morbidity or mortality
High volume or commonly occurring
Available options for prevention
Treatment available
Improved outcomes with early detection

The next and most important item is the case definition, which is an objective means of disease confirmation. The case definition may include a precise diagnostic test that is highly sensitive and/or specific. The case definition determines the numerator or top number in disease rate calculations. The target population determines the denominator or bottom number in disease rate calculations. Finally, determine how you will use the data collected. This will guide you and your team in the selection of the best type of surveillance activity.

Measures of Accuracy: Constructing Two-by-Two Tables

Earlier in this section we talked about describing the data set by using estimates of central tendency. The mean, median, and mode help you understand the data set without having to look at all of the data at once. Similarly, studies and their features can be described by a number of parameters that can be calculated from a 2 x 2 (read as "two-by-two") table. Before we define these parameters, let's look at the basic 2 x 2 table (see Table 13.7). You construct the 2 x 2 table by laying out the test result across the top and the condition or disease along the left hand side. Those patients who have the condition and have a positive test result are correctly identified by the test and are therefore truly positive (letter a), while those who have the condition but are not identified by the test are falsely negative (letter b). Similarly, those individuals who do not have the condition and are incorrectly identified by a positive test result are falsely positive (letter c), while those who do not have the condition and are not identified by the test are truly negative (letter d).

TABLE 13.7

The Basic 2 X 2 Table

		TEST RESULT		
		POSITIVE	NEGATIVE	TOTAL
Disease or Condition	Present	a	b	a+b
	Absent	c	d	c+d
	Total	a+c	b+d	a+b+c+d

a = true positive   b / a+b = false negative rate
b = false negative   c / c+d = false positive rate
c = false positive   a / a+c = positive predictive value
d = true negative   d / b+d = negative predictive value

Sensitivity and Specificity

The sensitivity of a test refers to the proportion of patients with the disease who have a positive test result. A perfect test gives a positive result for all patients who have the disease (van Stralen et al., 2009). Sensitivity is calculated by dividing the number of patients who are true positive (a) by the total number of patients with the disease (a + b). Tests that are sensitive are used to positively identify a disease or condition. A good test must accurately identify all those patients with the disease while testing negative for those patients who do not have the disease. The specificity of a test refers to the proportion of patients without the disease who have a negative test result. Specificity is calculated by dividing the number of patients who are true negative (d) by the total number of patients without the disease (c + d). Tests that are specific are used to exclude a disease or condition.

False Positive and False Negative Rates

The sensitivity and specificity can also be considered as the true positive and true negative rates, respectively. They tell you how good a test is at identifying or excluding a particular disease or condition. The false positive and false negative rates give you an idea of "how bad" tests are for identifying or excluding a particular disease or condition. The false positive rate is calculated by dividing the number of patients who are false positive (c) by the total number of patients without the disease (c + d). The false negative rate is calculated by dividing the number of patients who are false negative (b) by the total number of patients with the disease (a + b).

Positive Predictive Value and Negative Predictive Value

The positive predictive value of a test is the likelihood that the patient has the disease when looking at all positive test results. The positive predictive value of a test is calculated by dividing the number of positive test results in patients who are true positive (a) by the total number of positive test results (a + c). The negative predictive value of a test is the likelihood that the patient does not have the disease when looking at all negative test results. The negative predictive value of a test is calculated by dividing the number of negative test results in patients who are true negative (d) by the total number of negative test results (b + d).

Case Study 5: Use of Fever and Tonsillar Exudate and Lymphadenopathy to Identify Strep Throat

Now that John, Mary, and Susan understand some of the basic concepts of data collection and data analysis, they begin to think about their practice of patient care in a more meaningful way. At lunch one afternoon they talk with Dr. Wellbee about the number of rapid Strep tests that they need to keep in stock and ask how strep infection was diagnosed before these point of care tests were available. Dr. Wellbee tells them he relied on the clinical picture, and if fever, tonsillar exudates, and lymphadenopathy were present, he prescribed antibiotics because presence of this triad generally identified a case of Strep throat. The nurses decide to create a tracking tool (see Table 13.8). They collect data on all patients seen during the month of June and place the results in a data summary sheet (see Table 13.9). Dr. Wellbee instructs them to create a 2 x 2 table using the rapid strep test to identify those cases of Strep throat and the presence of all three features (fever, tonsillar exudate, and lymphadenopathy) as the clinical test being evaluated (see Table 13.10). He helps them calculate the sensitivity (22/31 = 71.0%), the specificity (17/19 = 89.5%), the positive predictive value (22/24 = 91.7%), and the negative predictive value (17/26 = 65.4%). Dr. Wellbee explains that the clinical test is highly specific—almost 90% of patients without the disease do not have all three clinical signs present. He also tells his nurses that the test has a high positive predictive value—almost 92% of patients with all three clinical signs have the disease.

TABLE 13.8
Strep Throat Tracking Tool

Patient Name:		
Date of Service:		
Fever	Y	N
Exudate	Y	N
Lymphadenopathy	Y	N
All Three	Y	N
Rapid Strep Test	Positive	Negative

TABLE 13.9
Strep Throat Data Summary Sheet

Data Collection Period:	June 1 to June 30	
Fever	Y = 40	N = 10
Exudate	Y = 32	N = 18
Lymphadenopathy	Y = 36	N = 14
All Three	Y = 24	N = 26
Rapid Strep Test	Y = 31	N = 19

TABLE 13.10

Strep Throat 2 x 2 Table

		CLINICAL TEST RESULT		
		POSITIVE	NEGATIVE	TOTAL
Strep Throat	Present	22	9	31
	Absent	2	17	19
	Total	24	26	50

COHORT STUDIES AND RELATIVE RISK

As we described earlier, a cohort study looks at a group of patients who have one or more common features. It is a form of a prospective study that helps us to study whether a particular risk factor is associated with a particular disease. The groups are matched for other variables so that the independent variable, the risk factor being studied, can be evaluated with regard to the dependant variable, the disease or condition. Cohort studies allow you to calculate the relative risk of acquiring the disease if the risk factor is present.

Case Study 7: Transmission of Methicillin-Resistant *Staphylococcus Aureus* (MRSA) in the Home Care Setting

Dr. Wellbee has noticed an increase in community-acquired MRSA in his middle and high school–aged students. He is concerned about the risk of transmission to other household members. He and his nurses decide to conduct a prospective study looking at all patients who test positive for MRSA and evaluate household members for disease transmission. They study 148 patients who are colonized with MRSA and 188 household contacts. They look at the following risk factors for household contacts: male gender, providing health care to the colonized patient, and sharing the same bedroom. They constructed Table 13.11. Dr. Wellbee helps his nurses construct a general relative risk table (see Table 13.12) as well as a specific one for this study. He explains that it is similar to the 2 x 2 table used to calculate sensitivity and specificity. Relative risk is calculated by dividing [a / (a + b)] by [c / (c + d)]. (See Table 13.13.)

Using the data provided, the relative risk equals (29/112) dividing by (7/76) or 2.82. Household contacts that provide health care to patients who are colonized with MRSA have 2.8 times the risk of acquiring MRSA compared to those household contacts that do not provide care. Given these data, Dr. Wellbee begins recommending that household contacts use similar infection control and prevention measures as those used in the hospital setting. (Adapted from Lucet et al., 2009.)

TABLE **13.11**

Household Acquisition of MRSA Data Table

CHARACTERISTIC	MRSA ACQUIRED (N=36)	MRSA NOT ACQUIRED (N=152)
Boys	13	71
Provides Health Care	29	83
Shares Bedroom	7	38

TABLE **13.12**

Generalized Relative Risk Table

	MRSA ACQUIRED	MRSA NOT ACQUIRED	TOTAL
Risk Factor Present	a	b	a+b
Risk Factor Absent	c	d	c+d
Total	a+c	b+d	a+b+c+d

TABLE **13.13**

Relative Risk of Household MRSA Acquisition for Members who Provide Direct Health Care

	MRSA ACQUIRED	MRSA NOT ACQUIRED	TOTAL
Provides Health Care	29	83	112
Does not Provide Health Care	7	69	76
Total	36	152	188

CASE CONTROL STUDIES AND ODDS RATIO

As described earlier, a case-control study is a retrospective, observational study that looks at patients with a similar condition (case) and compares them to similarly matched patients who do not have the condition (controls) to estimate the odds ratio between a risk factor and the development of a particular condition.

Case Study 8: Transmission of *Serratia Marcescens* Bloodstream Infection (BSI) from Contaminated, Pre-Filled Insulin Syringes

John, Mary, and Susan become concerned when several diabetic patients become hospitalized with Serratia BSI. They meet with Dr. Wellbee and decide they need to conduct a surveillance activity. They begin by interviewing some of the parents and learn that many have been using pre-filled insulin syringes provided by the local pharmacy. They create a data collection sheet that includes the use of pre-filled insulin syringes (see Table 13.14). They identify 162 diabetic patients and contact the local pharmacy and learn that 92 of them were receiving pre-filled insulin syringes. They create a data table. Dr. Wellbee then helps his nurses construct a general odds ratio table (see Table 13.15) as well as a specific one for this study. He explains that it is similar to the 2 x 2 table used to calculate sensitivity and specificity (see Table 13.16). The odds ratio is calculated by dividing [a x d] by [c x b]. Using the data provided in Table 13.17, the odds ratio equals (86 x 20) dividing by (50 x 6) or 5.73. Dr. Wellbee contacts the local department of health to investigate further and advises patients to stop using pre-filled insulin syringes. (Adapted from Blossom D, 2009.)

TABLE 13.14

Serratia BSI Associated with Pre-Filled Insulin Syringes Data Table

CHARACTERISTIC	BSI PRESENT (N=136)	BSI ABSENT (N=26)
Use of Pre-Filled Insulin Syringes	86	6

TABLE 13.15

Generalized Odds Ratio Table

	BSI PRESENT	BSI ABSENT	TOTAL
Risk Factor Present	a	b	a+b
Risk Factor Absent	c	d	c+d
Total	a+c	b+d	a+b+c+d

TABLE 13.16

Odds Ratio of Using Pre-Filled Insulin Syringes if Serratia BSI is Present

	SERRATIA BSI PRESENT	SERRATIA BSI ABSENT	TOTAL
Using Pre-Filled Insulin Syringes	86	6	92
Not Using Pre-Filled Insulin Syringes	50	20	70
Total	136	26	162

TABLE 13.17

Seasonal Influenza Status and Patient Age for Patients Seen on Friday April 2 and Cared For by Nurse Mary

NURSE	PATIENT AGE	VACCINE STATUS
Mary	1	Y
Mary	3	Y
Mary	3	Y
Mary	4	Y
Mary	6	N
Mary	9	N
Mary	9	N
Mary	13	N
Mary	13	N
Mary	14	N
Mary	14	N
Mary	15	N
Mary	15	N
Mary	18	N

THE PLAN, DO, CHECK, ACT (PDCA) CYCLE

Up until now we have focused on methods of acquiring and interpreting data in the context of surveillance. This represents the first step in the performance improvement process, which is often described as a multistep cycle, sometimes called the PDCA or Deming Cycle, named after William Edwards Deming who championed quality improvement. The PDCA cycle involves the establishment of a Plan (P), carrying out or Doing that plan (D), Checking or collecting more data (C), and then Acting on that data as needed (A).

The initial data set that is collected serves as your baseline. This must then be compared with local and/or national benchmarks. If it is determined that a problem exists, a root cause analysis (sometimes called a fish-bone diagram) should be performed. This addresses all possible explanations for the difference seen between your data and the benchmark comparator. The team then develops a corrective action plan based on the root cause analysis. This plan is put into place after which additional data are collected to determine if the desired improvement has occurred.

Case Study 9: Performance Improvement for Seasonal Influenza Vaccination

Dr. Wellbee is concerned about the risk of seasonal influenza in his patients. He reviews the data in Table 13.5 and focuses on the patients that Mary attended. He is troubled by the number and proportion of patients that are not vaccinated for seasonal influenza. Dr. Wellbee addresses this with Mary. She tells Dr. Wellbee that she often works with Dr. Geezer, who believes that "germs are good for you" and "what doesn't kill you will make the body strong." He doesn't believe in vaccination and as such doesn't offer it to his patients. He will, however, provide the vaccine if the patient or parent requests it. Dr. Wellbee and his nurses adopt a two-pronged approach that relies heavily on education. They bring in local influenza experts to provide education to all members of the office staff, both clinical as well as administrative. They segregate their waiting room into "well visit" and "sick visit," areas and they highlight this new design before and during flu season. They hang posters and place free patient handouts in the waiting and exam rooms. They coordinate seasonal influenza clinics and mail educational materials stressing the importance of vaccination along with invitations to patients and their families asking them to sign up for a flu shot. And maybe most importantly, Dr. Wellbee speaks to Dr. Geezer, informing him that he is not adhering to published guidelines and evidence-based medicine. One year later, seasonal influenza vaccination rates in Dr. Wellbee's patients exceed the national average.

SUMMARY

Surveillance should be part of every infection control and prevention program. It provides the data that helps guide and shape practice patterns in order to minimize risks and optimize patient care.

POST-TEST QUESTIONS

13-1. Which of the following types of surveillance relies on data collected from a subset of the population that can then be generalized back to the broader population?

     a. Administrative surveillance
     b. Vector surveillance
     c. Laboratory-based surveillance
     d. Sentinel surveillance

13-2. What is calculated by adding the list of values and dividing by the number of values in the data set?
     a. Mean
     b. Median
     c. Mode
     d. Benchmark

13-3. What study type identifies all cases by "looking backward" using a chart review?
     a. Longitudinal
     b. Cross-sectional
     c. Prospective
     d. Retrospective

13-4. Which of the following refers to the proportion of patients with the disease who have a positive test result?
     a. Specificity
     b. Sensitivity
     c. Positive predictive value
     d. Negative predictive value

13-5. What does the "D" stand for in the PDCA cycle?
     a. Debate
     b. Discover
     c. Do
     d. Deliver

References

Blossom, D., Noble-Wang, J., Su, J., Pur, S., Chemaly, R., Shams, A., et al. (2009). Multistate outbreak of Serratia marcescens bloodstream infections caused by contamination of prefilled heparin and isotonic sodium chloride solution syringes. *Archives of Internal Medicine, 169,* 1705–1711.

Gastmeier, P., Coignard, B., & Horan, T. (2007). Surveillance for healthcare associated infections. In N.M. M'ikanatha, R. Lynfield, C.A. Van Beneden, & H. de Valk (Eds.), *Infectious disease surveillance* (pp. 159–170). Malden, MA: Blackwell Publishing.

Lucet, J.C., Paoletti, X., Demontpion, C., Degrave, M., Vanjak, D., Vincent, C., et al. (2009). Carriage of methicillin-resistant Staphylococcus aureus in home care settings. *Archives of Internal Medicine, 169,* 1372–1378.

M'ikanatha, N.M., Lynfield, R., Julian, K.G., Van Beneden, C.A., & de Valk, H. (2007). Infectious disease surveillance: A cornerstone for prevention and control. In N. M'ikanatha, R. Lynfield, C.A. Van Beneden, & H. de Valk (Eds.), *Infectious disease surveillance* (pp. 3–17). Malden, MA: Blackwell Publishing.

van Stralen, K.J., Stel, V.S., Reitsma, J.B., Dekker, F.W., Zoccali, C., & Jager, K.J. (2009). Diagnostic methods I: sensitivity, specificity, and other measures of accuracy. *Kidney International, 75,* 1257–1263.

Weisstein, E.W. (n.d.). Normal distribution. *Mathworld.* Retrieved January 31, 2010, from http://mathworld.wolfram.com/NormalDistribution.html

Influenza

14

This chapter includes the identification of the patient population at highest risk for developing severe illness and complications from the influenza virus. Vaccine recommendations and contraindications and precautions of vaccine are reviewed. The content differentiates between the two types of influenza viruses, type A and type B. There is also discussion on H1N1 influenza.

OBJECTIVES

1. Identify the patient population at highest risk for developing severe illness and complications from the influenza virus.
2. Define the age(s) of the patient population that the influenza vaccine should be offered.
3. Discuss the role of the visiting nurse in the administration of the influenza vaccine.
4. Discuss the recommendations for providing the influenza vaccine to patients who reside in nursing homes or long-term care residential facilities.
5. Explain the rationale for health care providers to be encouraged to receive the influenza vaccine.

PRE-TEST QUESTIONS

14-1. Which of the following best describes the method of transmission for influenza infection?
   a. Droplet transmission
   b. Bloodborne transmission
   c. Sexual transmission
   d. Contact transmission
14-2. Which of the following is a common symptom of influenza?
   a. Malaise
   b. Renal failure
   c. Jaundice
   d. Meningitis

14-3. Which of the following children is considered high risk for influenza complications and should be vaccinated with the influenza vaccine?
  a. A 10-month-old child
  b. A 16 year old with hypertension
  c. A 12 year old with diabetes
  d. All of the above

14-4. The inactive influenza vaccine:
  a. Is administered through the nose
  b. Is a live virus vaccine
  c. Can only be administered to people between the ages of 6 months and 49 years
  d. Can be administered to individuals who are at high risk for medical complications associated with influenza infection

14-5. Which of the following patients should not receive any type of influenza vaccine?
  a. A patient with a history of anaphylaxis to eggs
  b. A patient with an upper respiratory tract infection
  c. A pregnant woman
  d. A 9-month-old child

The two types of influenza viruses that cause widespread human disease are influenza A and influenza B. The virus is spread from person-to-person primarily through droplet transmission. Patients sometimes confuse the signs and symptoms of the common cold and influenza. Signs and symptoms of the influenza virus include fever, myalgia, headache, malaise, nonproductive cough, sore throat, and rhinitis. Following are signs and symptoms of the common cold versus seasonal or H1N1 influenza.

Differentiating Cold and Influenza

H1N1 or Seasonal Flu Symptoms

- Fever
- More painful body aches
- Dry cough
- Diarrhea
- Severe fatigue
- Respiratory problems
- Dehydration

Cold Symptoms

- Stuffy nose
- Congestion
- Body aches
- Growing cough
- Symptoms last 3 to 5 days

In the United States, the influenza season typically occurs during the fall or winter months. This is when most of the annual outbreaks of the virus occur.

However, infection with influenza virus can occur as late as April or May. Infection with influenza virus has the potential to lead to severe illnesses that may result in hospitalizations or even deaths. The patient population at the highest risk for developing severe illnesses from influenza are children younger than 2 years, adults 65 years or older, and people of any age group with certain pre-existing medical conditions.

In 2009, it was recommended that children aged 6 months to 18 years receive the flu vaccine if they meet any of the conditions listed in Table 14.1.

Note that children aged less than 6 months cannot receive influenza vaccination. Household and other close contacts (e.g., daycare providers) of children aged less than 6 months, including older children and adolescents, should be vaccinated.

The 2009 adult flu vaccine recommendations are also listed in Table 14.1.

TABLE 14.1

Seasonal Influenza Vaccination Recommendations 2009

6 months to 18 years	Adults
Have chronic pulmonary (including asthma), cardiovascular (except hypertension), renal, hepatic, cognitive, neurologic/neuromuscular, hematological, or metabolic disorders (including diabetes mellitus)	Persons aged ≥50 years
Are immunosuppressed (including immunosuppression caused by medications or by human immunodeficiency virus)	Women who will be pregnant during the influenza season
Are receiving long-term aspirin therapy and therefore might be at risk for experiencing Reye syndrome after influenza virus infection	Persons who have chronic pulmonary (including asthma), cardiovascular (except hypertension), renal, hepatic, cognitive, neurologic/neuromuscular, hematological, or metabolic disorders (including diabetes mellitus)
Are residents of long-term care facilities	Persons who have immunosuppression (including immunosuppression caused by medications or by HIV)
Will be pregnant during the influenza season	Residents of nursing homes and other long-term care facilities
	Health care personnel
	Household contacts and caregivers of children aged <5 years and adults aged ≥50 years, with particular emphasis on vaccinating contacts of children aged <6 months
	Household contacts and caregivers of persons with medical conditions that put them at higher risk for severe complications from influenza.

From Centers for Disease Control and Prevention [CDC], 2009.

According to the CDC there are three preventative actions to combat influenza. These include vaccination, appropriate hygiene, and antiviral medications. There are two different types of influenza virus vaccine available in the United States: live, attenuated influenza vaccine (LAIV) and inactivated influenza vaccine (TIV; see Table 14.2).

TABLE **14.2**

Live, Attenuated Influenza Vaccine (LAIV) Compared with Inactivated Influenza Vaccine (TIV) for Seasonal Influenza, U.S. Formulations

FACTOR	LAIV	TIV
Route of administration	Intranasal spray	Intramuscular injection
Type of vaccine	Live virus	Noninfectious virus (i.e., inactivated)
No. of included virus strains	Three (two influenza A, one influenza B)	Three (two influenza A, one influenza B)
Vaccine virus strains updated	Annually	Annually
Frequency of administration	Annually[a]	Annually[a]
Approved age	Persons aged 2–49 yrs[†]	Persons aged $\geq$6 mos
Interval between 2 doses recommended for children aged $\geq$6 mos to 8 yrs who are receiving influenza vaccine for the first time	4 wks	4 wks
Can be administered to persons with medical risk factors for influenza-related complications[†]	No	Yes
Can be administered to children with asthma or children aged 2–4 yrs with wheezing in the past year[§]	No	Yes
Can be administered to family members or close contacts of immunosuppressed persons not requiring a protected environment	Yes	Yes
Can be administered to family members or close contacts of immunosuppressed persons requiring a protected environment (e.g., hematopoietic stem cell transplant recipient)	No	Yes

(*Continued*)

TABLE 14.2

(Continued)

FACTOR	LAIV	TIV
Can be administered to family members or close contacts of persons at high risk but not severely immunosuppressed	Yes	Yes
Can be simultaneously administered with other vaccines	Yes	Yes**
If not simultaneously administered, can be administered within 4 wks of another live vaccine	Space 4 wks apart	Yes
If not simultaneously administered, can be administered within 4 wks of an inactivated vaccine	Yes	Yes

Notes: Children aged 6 months to 8 years who have never received influenza vaccine before should receive two doses. Those who only receive one dose in their first year of vaccination should receive two doses in the following year, spaced 4 weeks apart.

Persons at higher risk for complications of influenza infection because of underlying medical conditions should not receive LAIV. Persons at higher risk for complications of influenza infection because of underlying medical conditions include adults and children with chronic disorders of the pulmonary or cardiovascular systems; adults and children with chronic metabolic diseases (including diabetes mellitus), renal dysfunction, hemoglobinopathies, or immunosuppression; children and adolescents receiving long-term aspirin therapy (at risk for developing Reye syndrome after wild-type influenza infection); persons who have any condition (e.g., cognitive dysfunction, spinal cord injuries, seizure disorders, or other neuromuscular disorders) that can compromise respiratory function or the handling of respiratory secretions or that can increase the risk for aspiration; pregnant women; and residents of nursing homes and other chronic-care facilities that house persons with chronic medical conditions.

Clinicians and immunization programs should screen for possible reactive airway diseases when considering use of LAIV for children aged 2–4 years and should avoid use of this vaccine in children with asthma or a recent wheezing episode. Health care providers should consult the medical record, when available, to identify children aged 2–4 years with asthma or recurrent wheezing that might indicate asthma. In addition, to identify children who might be at greater risk for asthma and possibly at increased risk for wheezing after receiving LAIV, parents or caregivers of children aged 2–4 years should be asked: "In the past 12 months, has a health care provider ever told you that your child had wheezing or asthma?" Children whose parents or caregivers answer "yes" to this question and children who have asthma or who had a wheezing episode noted in the medical record during the preceding 12 months should not receive LAIV.

LAIV coadministration has been evaluated systematically only among children aged 12–15 months who received measles, mumps, and rubella vaccine or varicella vaccine.

* aTIV coadministration has been evaluated systematically only among adults who received pneumococcal polysaccharide or zoster vaccine.

From "Prevention and Control of Seasonal Influenza—Recommendations of the Advisory Committee on Immunization Practices (ACIP)," by Centers for Disease Control and Prevention, 2009. *MMWR, 58*(RR08), 1–52.

There are a number of contraindications and precautions to consider when administering the influenza vaccine. Contraindications and precautions are listed in Table 14.3 (Advisory Committee on Immunization Practices [ACIP], Vaccines for Children Program, 2008).

It is not necessary to obtain a formal signed consent prior to administration of the influenza vaccination. However, patients should be educated regarding general vaccine information as well as the benefits and risks of being vaccinated. All patients should receive the most updated vaccine information statement (VIS) every time they receive the immunization.

ACUTE-CARE HOSPITALS

Acute-care hospitals have a responsibility to protect hospitalized patients from the influenza virus. It is important to obtain patients' influenza vaccination history on admission and, if indicated, to administer the vaccine during the hospitalization. The vaccination of inpatients is usually facilitated through the use of hospital-specific standing orders. During hospitalization, the influenza vaccine

TABLE 14.3

Contraindications and Precautions of Influenza Vaccine (TIV or LAIV)

CONTRAINDICATIONS	PRECAUTIONS
Allergy to vaccine components	History of Guillain-Barre' Syndrome (GBS) following influenza vaccination
Moderate or severe illnesses with or without fever	

Contraindications and Precautions to Administration of LAIV

CONTRAINDICATIONS	PRECAUTIONS
Concomitant aspirin therapy	<24 months of age
	Asthma/recurrent wheezing
	Altered immunocompetence
	Medical conditions predisposing to Influenza Complications
	Pregnant women

From "Prevention and Control of Seasonal Influenza—Recommendations of the Advisory Committee on Immunization Practices (ACIP)," by Centers for Disease Control and Prevention, 2009. MMWR, 58(RR08), 1–52.

should be offered to those at high risk. Standing orders to offer influenza vaccination to all hospitalized persons should be considered.

VISITING NURSES PROVIDING HOME CARE

During influenza season, visiting nurses that provide home care to patients should identify patients who are eligible for the influenza vaccine and administer the vaccine if indicated. Household members of high-risk patients should also be encouraged by the visiting nurse to get vaccinated for influenza.

NURSING HOMES AND OTHER RESIDENTIAL LONG-TERM–CARE FACILITIES

It is important to routinely provide the influenza vaccination to patients who reside in nursing homes or other residential long-term care facilities. These patients should be vaccinated prior to the influenza season or as soon as the vaccine becomes available to the facility. In addition, all residents who are newly admitted to the facility during influenza season should be offered the vaccine.

All facilities that accept Medicare and Medicaid insurance plans have additional requirements to follow. The Centers for Medicare and Medicaid Services (CMS) require that all eligible residents must be offered the influenza vaccine. CMS also requires that the vaccine administration and history must be documented in the resident's medical records. The only conditions acceptable for a resident to not receive the vaccine are a medical contraindication to the vaccine, a refusal of the vaccine by the resident or a legal representative, or the unavailability of the vaccine due to a shortage.

HEALTH CARE WORKERS (HCWS)

HCWs should be offered the influenza vaccination during influenza season due to their increased risk of exposure to the influenza virus as well as the risk of transmitting the virus to the patients for whom they are responsible. Employee education should emphasize the importance of obtaining an influenza vaccine to help protect themselves and their patients from influenza infection. Education should also include the benefits and risks of the vaccine as well as the potential harmful effects and complications of the influenza virus. Health care facilities should consider providing influenza vaccination campaigns so employees have convenient access to the immunization.

THE H1N1 FLU

Novel H1N1 (initially called "swine flu") is a novel influenza virus causing influenza infection in people. This virus was first detected in people in the United

States in April 2009. This virus spreads from person to person, probably in much the same way that regular seasonal influenza viruses spread. On June 11, 2009, the World Health Organization (WHO) signaled that a pandemic of novel H1N1 flu was underway.

The symptoms of H1N1 flu in people are similar to the symptoms of seasonal influenza and include fever, cough, sore throat, body aches, headache, chills, and fatigue. Some people have reported diarrhea and vomiting associated with H1N1 flu. In the past, severe illness (pneumonia and respiratory failure) and deaths have been reported with H1N1 flu infection in people. Like seasonal flu, H1N1 flu may cause a worsening of underlying chronic medical conditions.

A vaccine for the H1N1 flu has recently been approved by the Food and Drug Administration (FDA), but this is an evolving area. For the most updated information on the H1N1 flu vaccine, see http://www.flu.gov

POST-TEST QUESTIONS

14-1. Which of the following best describes the method of transmission for influenza infection?
   a. Droplet transmission
   b. Bloodborne transmission
   c. Sexual transmission
   d. Contact transmission

14-2. Which of the following is a common symptom of influenza?
   a. Malaise
   b. Renal failure
   c. Jaundice
   d. Meningitis

14-3. Which of the following children is considered high risk for influenza complications and should be vaccinated with the influenza vaccine?
   a. A 10-month-old child
   b. A 16 year old with hypertension
   c. A 12 year old with diabetes
   d. All of the above

14-4. The inactive influenza vaccine:
   a. Is administered through the nose
   b. Is a live virus vaccine
   c. Can only be administered to people between the ages of 6 months and 49 years
   d. Can be administered to individuals who are at high risk for medical complications associated with influenza infection

14-5. Which of the following patients should not receive any type of influenza vaccine?
   a. A patient with a history of anaphylaxis to eggs
   b. A patient with an upper respiratory tract infection
   c. A pregnant woman
   d. A 9-month-old child

References

Advisory Committee on Immunization Practices, Vaccines for Children Program. (2008). *Vaccines to prevent influenza.* Retrieved September 1, 2009, from http://www.cdc.gov/vaccines/programs/vfc/down loads/resolutions/0208influenza.pdf

Centers for Disease Control and Prevention. (2009). Prevention and control of seasonal influenza—Recommendations of the Advisory Committee on Immunization Practices (ACIP). *MMWR, 58*(RR08), 1–52. Retrieved September 1, 2009, from http://www.cdc.gov/mmwr/PDF/rr/rr5808.pdf

Tuberculosis

15

This chapter includes a discussion of the primary method of transmission of *Mycobacterium tuberculosis* (TB). The content differentiates between latent and active tuberculosis. The four signs and symptoms of mycobacterium tuberculosis infection are reviewed. There is discussion on miliary TB and Mantoux testing. Finally, methods used to prevent the transmission of TB are discussed.

OBJECTIVES

1. List the primary method of transmission of mycobacterium tuberculosis.
2. Explain the difference between latent tuberculosis and active tuberculosis
3. Identify four signs and symptoms of mycobacterium tuberculosis infection.
4. Explain the testing procedures used to diagnose tuberculosis infection.
5. Identify methods used to prevent the transmission of tuberculosis.

PRE-TEST QUESTIONS

15-1. Tuberculosis infection is caused by a(n):
   a. Virus
   b. Bacteria
   c. Parasite
   d. Amoeba
15-2. Tuberculosis is spread to another person by:
   a. Airborne droplets
   b. Sexual contact
   c. Contaminated medical equipment
   d. Exposure to contaminated bed linens
15-3. Symptoms commonly seen in a patient with tuberculosis include:
   a. High, spiking fever
   b. Weight gain due to fluid retention
   c. Coughing
   d. Constipation
15-4. When administering a purified protein derivative (PPD) test for tuberculosis, which of the following is FALSE?

a. A small amount of a substance called PPD (purified protein derivative) tuberculin is injected intradermally inside the forearm.

b. As the solution is injected a definite pale bleb (wheal) should appear.

c. A tight dressing is applied to the intradermal injection site.

d. The site of injection is visually checked by a health care professional
48–72 hours after injection.

15-5. Which of the following medications is commonly used in the prevention
and treatment of tuberculosis?

a. Amoxicillin

b. Isoniazid

c. Zidovudine

d. Chloroquine

Tuberculosis (TB) is caused by a bacterium, *Mycobacterium tuberculosis*
(MTB; see Figure 15.1). Evidence of TB disease has been discovered in the bones
thought to be of a mother and baby, excavated from Alit-Yam, a 9,000-year-old
Pre-Pottery Neolithic village that had been submerged off the coast of Haifa, Is-
rael, for thousands of years.

Early names for TB, such as "consumption" and "white plague," were evidence
that TB infection was considered a death sentence. Early treatment in the United
States meant isolation. The poor were sent to tent cities in Arizona or taken by
authorities to overcrowded hospitals. Children were removed from families.

Those who could afford to travel went to sanitariums in the mountains, sometimes for years. The cold, clear air, rest, and good nutrition were believed to heal
the lungs. Most of the time the treatment not only helped cure the disease but

FIGURE 15.1

Microscopic view of
Mycobacterium tuberculosis

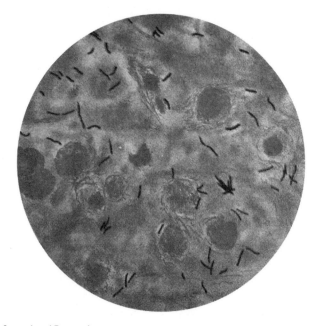

Courtesy of the Centers for Disease Control and Prevention.

also stopped it from spreading. In 1943, the first antibiotic effective against TB, streptomycin, was developed and doctors had something to fight TB. The mortality rate began to drop. Improved living conditions, early diagnosis, and treatment made TB an almost exhausted disease by the 1960s. In fact, the Centers for Disease Control and Prevention (CDC) issued "A Strategic Plan for the Elimination of Tuberculosis in the United States" in 1988. It was hoped that by 2010, TB would be eradicated (CDC, 1989, pp. 1–25). Unfortunately, by the early 1990s that hope had faded. In 1991, there was an increase in new cases of TB, and this number grew annually. An epidemic was in the making. Larger numbers of poverty-stricken people living in crowed, unhealthy areas were susceptible. This included minorities, mentally ill and the elderly, and patients with AIDS. Another disturbing finding was that MTB seemed able to mutate more rapidly than previously believed and developed a rapid resistance to antibiotics. Streptomycin was not effective in all cases.

TRANSMISSION

TB travels person to person through airborne particle from the respiratory track, which occurs when an infected person coughs, sneezes, talks, or sings (Figure 15.2). The transmission occurs when the particles enter the respiratory track of the noninfected person. Casual contact with an infected person usually does not result in transmission of the disease; prolonged contact is usually needed. If transmission has occurred, symptoms may not develop for years.

There are many factors that contribute to the transmission of TB in the United States and worldwide.

- *Crowed living conditions.* The illness easily transfers from person to person in cramped, poorly ventilated spaces like prisons, juvenile detention centers, and shelters for the homeless. Extended care facilities are also an area of high transmission as older adults have weakened immune systems from age or illness.
- *Increased numbers of foreign-born nationals.* The TB rates for people born in the United States are declining; the rates among people from other parts of the world are increasing.
- *Increased poverty and lack of access to medical care.* The poor in the United States and around the world are more likely to have TB and less likely to receive medical care. The problem becomes worse because people living in poverty often move or migrate, and therefore may not complete their treatment, leading to drug-resistant forms of the disease.
- *Increase in drug resistant strains of TB.* There is a TB strain that will resist each major TB medication made. Even more worrisome are strains that are resistant to at least two anti-TB drugs, leading to multidrug-resistant tuberculosis (MDR-TB). People carrying MDR-TB are highly contagious with these super-TB bacteria.

As the infection is primarily transmitted through the air, there is virtually no danger of contracting the illness through dishes, linens, or other items touched

FIGURE 15.2

Pattern of airborne droplet formation after a sneeze

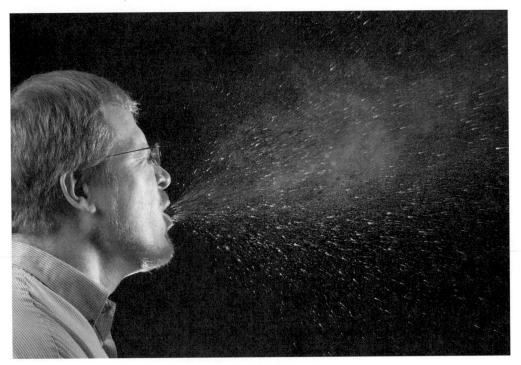

Courtesy of the Centers for Disease Control and Prevention / Brian Judd.

by someone infected with TB. Sometimes TB can be transmitted through some food products, such as unpasteurized milk or milk products (some cheeses) obtained from infected cattle (CDC, 2009).

The emergence of drug-resistant strains of the bacterium that cause the disease, along with HIV/AIDS, poverty, and the lack of health services, have made world-wide infection common. Approximately one-third of the human population is infected, with some parts of the population at a higher risk for infection. More than one-fourth of the reported TB cases in the United States occur in people older than 65.

RATE OF TB CASES, BY STATE—UNITED STATES, 2006

Additionally, according to 2006 CDC statistics, more cases of TB were reported among Hispanics than among any other ethnic population in the United States. At this time in the United States, two-thirds of all TB cases affect African Americans, Hispanics, Asians, and people from the Pacific Islands. Another one-fourth of TB cases in the United States occur in people born in another country (CDC, 2007).

TABLE 15.1

Differentiating Latent TB Infection From Active TB Infection

A PERSON WITH LATENT TB INFECTION	A PERSON WITH ACTIVE TB DISEASE
▓ Has no symptoms	▓ Has symptoms that may include: - a bad cough that lasts 3 weeks or longer - pain in the chest - coughing up blood or sputum - weakness or fatigue - weight loss - no appetite - chills - fever - sweating at night
▓ Does not feel sick	▓ Usually feels sick
▓ Cannot spread TB bacteria to others	▓ May spread TB bacteria to others
▓ Usually has a skin test or blood test result indicating TB infection	▓ Usually has a skin test or blood test result indicating TB infection
▓ Has a normal chest x-ray and a negative sputum smear	▓ May have an abnormal chest x-ray, or positive sputum smear or culture
▓ Needs treatment for latent TB infection to prevent active TB disease	▓ Needs treatment to treat active TB disease

SIGNS AND SYMPTOMS

Although the body may harbor the TB bacteria, a healthy immune system can prevent the development of TB disease. The immune system begins to attack the TB bacteria 2 to 8 weeks after infection occurs. Sometimes the bacteria do not die and remain in an inactive state known as latent TB infection (LTBI), causing no symptoms, and sometimes TB disease may develop (see Table 15.1).

TB mainly affects the lungs (pulmonary TB), and coughing is often the first and only symptom. Other signs and symptoms of active pulmonary TB include low grade fever, anorexia, unintended weight loss, night sweats, chills, pleurisy, lethargy, and dyspnea.

While TB affects primarily the lungs, it can spread to other parts of the body. In extrapulmonary TB the symptoms may be more severe. The signs and symptoms vary depending on the organs involved. TB of the spine may result in back pain, while TB that affects the kidneys might cause hematuria. Additionally, the pericardium, joints, meninges, lymph nodes, and the pleural space can be involved.

Miliary TB is a widespread dissemination of MTB. It may occur in one organ (5%), in several organs, or throughout the entire body (>90%) including the brain. Miliary TB is characterized by a large amount of TB bacilli that are smaller than those usually found and can easily be missed. If untreated, it is fatal. It may be difficult to diagnose because miliary TB can mimic many diseases. A high index of clinical suspicion is important to obtain an early diagnosis and start treatment.

TESTING PROCEDURES

A simple skin test, called a Mantoux test or TB skin test (TST), remains the most commonly used diagnostic tool to test for TB.

For this test a small amount of a substance called purified protein derivative (PPD) tuberculin is injected intradermally inside the forearm (see Figure 15.3).

As the solution is injected a definite pale bleb or wheal appears. The bleb will disperse within minutes. No pressure or dressing is needed. The site of injection is visually checked by a health care professional 48 to 72 hours after injection. Depending on the response, the test is diagnosed as positive or negative. A positive response will usually be shown as a hard, raised lump or induration at the injection site and indicates a tuberculosis infection (see Figure 15.4).

False positive or false negative results can occur with the TST. A false positive test suggests the presence of TB when it is actually not present. This can happen following exposure to a mycobacterium bacteria other than the one that causes TB, or if you have received a vaccine called bacillus Calmette-Guerin or BCG. BCG is a vaccine rarely given in the United States, but it is still used in countries with high rates of TB infection. A false negative test may occur under several circumstances.

Reasons for False Negative TB Skin Test

- Recent TB infection. It can take 8 to 10 weeks for the body to react after becoming infected.
- Severely weakened immune system. If the immune system is weakened by an illness, such as HIV, or by chemotherapy drugs, the Mantoux test may not cause a response even though TB is present.
- Vaccination with a live virus. If you receive a vaccine that contains a live virus like smallpox or measles it can interfere with the Mantoux test.

FIGURE 15.3

Intradermal administration of a TB test

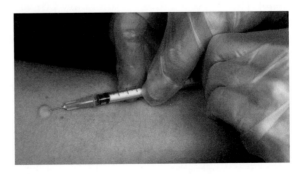

Courtesy of the Centers for Disease Control and Prevention / Gabrielle Benenson. Photo by Greg Knobloch.

FIGURE 15.4

Interpreting a TB test

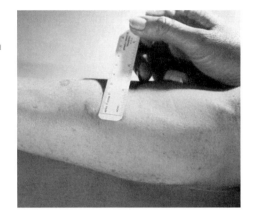

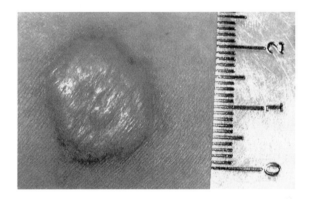

- Overwhelming TB disease. If TB has overwhelmed the body, it may not be possible for the body to produce a response.
- Improper testing. If the PPD tuberculin is injected too deeply below the surface of the skin the reaction may not be visible.

Newer methods of diagnosing the presence of TB are available but not routinely used. The QuantiFERON®-TB Gold or QFT test is an FDA-approved diagnostic aid that uses whole blood samples that are mixed with antigens and controls. After incubation for 16 to 24 hours the amount of interferon-gamma (IFN-gamma) is measured. If the patient is infected with MTB, their WBCs will release IFN-gamma in response to contact with TB antigens. Researchers are also investigating another test used primarily in developing countries, the microscopic-observation drug-susceptibility (MODS) assay. This test relies on sputum samples to detect the presence of TB bacteria. It can also identify drug-resistant strains of the bacteria. The MODS produces very accurate results in approximately one week.

If the results of a TB test are positive, further tests are needed to determine if LTBI or TB disease is present. These may include a chest x-ray, which could

FIGURE FIGURE 15.5

Chest x-ray of a patient with pulmonary tuberculosis

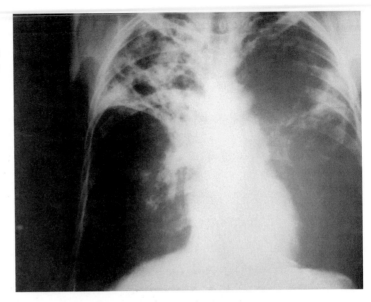

Courtesy of the Centers for Disease Control and Prevention.

indicate the presence of active pulmonary TB or show granulomata or white spots where your immune system has walled off TB bacteria or culture tests (Figure 15.5). If the chest x-ray or a urine sample indicates the signs of TB infection, then samples from the stomach or lung secretions are collected and stained for TB bacteria. These results are usually available in hours.

Travelers who think they may have been exposed or have spent an extended period of time in an endemic country should have a baseline test done. If the results are negative, then annual screening would identify recent infection, which would prompt medical evaluation.

TREATMENT

People who are infected with MTB can be treated to prevent progression to TB disease. The CDC recommends 6–9 months of isoniazid (INH) for the treatment of uncomplicated LTBI. Isoniazid is the preferred treatment, but 4 months of rifampin is a reasonable alternative (CDC, 2010).

In cases of TB disease, hospitalization may be needed for 2 weeks until tests indicate that the patient is no longer contagious. Four medications are recommended with a diagnosis of TB disease—isoniazid, rifampin, ethambutol, and pyrazinamide. If susceptibility tests show some of these drugs to be ineffective the wregimen may change. Some of these drugs have been combined into a single tablet, making the therapy less complicated, while making sure that MTB is destroyed. Although uncommon, long-term exposure to these drugs may be associated with a variety of side effects, including liver disease, which makes physician monitoring very important during treatment. Patients should also be instructed to avoid the use of acetaminophen (e.g., Tylenol, others) and to avoid or greatly limit alcohol consumption; both of which may greatly increase the risk of liver damage. Patients also need to be instructed to call their physician with any of the following:

- Nausea or vomiting
- Loss of appetite
- jaundice
- A fever lasting 3 or more days without obvious cause
- Abdominal tenderness or pain
- Color blindness or blurred vision

When hospitalization is necessary many techniques are used to prevent cross contamination. Patients with TB disease are isolated for approximately 2 weeks. Isolation rooms are used for patients with either a diagnosis of TB disease or a suspicion of having the disease. Isolation rooms are under negative pressure, which are designed to bring fresh air into the room. These rooms need exhaust vents that lead directly to the outside and must be placed away from intake vents. High efficiency particulate air (HEPA) filters and ultraviolet light are an alternative to negative pressure rooms. Portable HEPA air filter units recirculate room air and effectively remove all particles from the air in the size range of droplet nuclei. The filters must be properly designed, installed, and maintained. Those responsible for maintaining and handling the used filters should wear a respirator, eye protection, and gloves as the risk for handling contaminated filters has not been evaluated.

Any patient with a cough should be given a surgical mask until the reason for cough has been determined or until TB has been excluded as the cause. All staff in close contact need to be protected. The employer must have a respiratory protection program in place; most are presently using the N95 respirator.

The mask must fit snug to the face, making it impossible for airborne microorganisms to be inhaled. Facial hair and facial features may prevent a proper fit. The N95 medical grade mask (respirator) is designed to filter out viral pathogens and protect the nose and mouth in a pandemic environment (OSHA standard 29 CFR 1910.134).

Hospitalization is not the only means of isolation, but strict measures must be maintained if the patient is allowed to be in isolation at home. To minimize the chance of spreading TB, the infected person must stay at home, ensure adequate ventilation, and cover their mouth when coming in contact with others. Although treatment regimens are lengthy and associated with adverse effects, it is the only method that results in eradication of TB disease.

PREVENTION

Generally, TB is a preventable disease. Health care workers (HCWs) are continually fighting to prevent the spread of infection. There are measures that the general population can take to help protect themselves and others. Patients should be counseled to maintain healthy eating habits, exercise regularly, and get adequate amounts of sleep. Immunosuppressed patients, HCWs, and those working in a prison or nursing home should consider preventive therapy in the case of LTBI. Under these circumstances, therapy would reduce the risk of developing the disease in the future.

TB can be prevented and treated. Unfortunately, scientists have not been able to eradicate this devastating illness, which kills nearly 2 million people worldwide annually. Despite great advancement in the treatment of TB, it remains a global pandemic.

POST-TEST QUESTIONS

15-1. Tuberculosis infection is caused by a(n):
   a. Virus
   b. Bacteria
   c. Parasite
   d. Amoeba

15-2. Tuberculosis is spread to another person by:
   a. Airborne droplets
   b. Sexual contact
   c. Contaminated medical equipment
   d. Exposure to contaminated bed linens

15-3. Symptoms commonly seen in a patient with tuberculosis include:
   a. High, spiking fever
   b. Weight gain due to fluid retention
   c. Coughing
   d. Constipation

15-4. When administering a purified protein derivative (PPD) test for tuberculosis, which of the following is FALSE?
   a. A small amount of a substance called PPD (purified protein derivative) tuberculin is injected intradermally inside the forearm.
   b. As the solution is injected a definite pale bleb (wheal) should appear.
   c. A tight dressing is applied to the intradermal injection site.
   d. The site of injection is visually checked by a health care professional 48–72 hours after injection.

15-5. Which of the following medications is commonly used in the prevention and treatment of tuberculosis?
   a. Amoxicillin
   b. Isoniazid
   c. Zidovudine
   d. Chloroquine

References

Centers for Disease Control and Prevention. (1989). A strategic plan for the elimination of tuberculosis in the United States. *MMWR, 38,* 1–25.

Centers for Disease Control and Prevention. (2007). Trends in tuberculosis incidence—United States, 2006. *MMWR, 56*(11), 245–250. Retrieved August 13, 2007, from http:www.cdc.gov/mmwr/preview/mmwrhtml/mm5611a2.htm

Centers for Disease Control and Prevention. (2009). Chapter 5: Other infectious diseases related to travel. Retrieved November, 4, 2008, from http://www.cdc.gov/print.do?url=http%3A//wwwn.cdc.gov/travel/yellowBookCH4-TB.aspx

Centers for Disease Control and Prevention. (2010). Treatment of latent tuberculosis infection. Retrieved from www.cdc.gov/tb/publications/factsheets/treatment/treatmentLTBI.htm

Mayo Clinic Staff. (2009). *Tuberculosis*. Retrieved November 3, 2008, from http://www.mayoclinic.com/print/tuberculosis/DS00372/METHOD=print&DSECTION=all

Occupational Safety & Health Administration. (n.d.). Standard 29 CFR 1910.134.

Web Sites

http://www.emedicine.com/PED/topic2321.htm 11/3/08

http://www.cdc.gov/mmwr/preview/mmwrhtml/00001897.htm 12/30/08

http://www.medicalnewstoday.com/articles/119588.php 1/2/09

http://www.medicalnewstoday.com/articles/125562.php 1/2/09

http://www.cdc.gov/tb/pubs/tbfactsheet/BCG.htm 11/4/08

http://www.cdc.gov/vaccines/vpd-vac/tb/photos.htm 11/4/08

http://www.medicinenet.com/tuberculosis/index.htm 11/4/08

http://www.mayoclinic.com/print/tuberculosis/DS00372/METHOD=print&DSECTION=all 11/3/08

http://.fluarmour.com/proddetail.php?prod=FA111&gclid=CIvO96n)6pYCFQikHg . . . 11/10/08

16

Antibiotic-Resistant Infections

This chapter includes topics on the methods to reduce the development of antibiotic resistance. The content items include: methicillin-resistant *S. aureus* and *vancomycin-resistant enterococci*. There is discussion on the reduction of incidence of *C. difficile*–associated disease.

OBJECTIVES

1. List three methods to reduce the development of antibiotic resistance.
2. Name two antibiotics that can be used in patients with methicillin-resistant *S. aureus* infection.
3. List three risk factors for the development of an infection due to vancomycin-resistant enterococci.
4. Describe two methods of reducing the incidence of *C. difficile*–associated disease.

PRE-TEST QUESTIONS

16-1. Which of the following bacteria are associated with antibiotic resistance?
   a. *Staphylococcus aureus*
   b. Enterococci
   c. *Clostridium difficile*
   d. All of the above

16-2. One of the most important measures of control of antibiotic resistance is:
   a. Judicious use of antibiotics
   b. Hepatitis C infections

      c. Increasing number of viral infections

      d. All of the above

16-3. Overuse of which of the following antibiotics has been associated with antibiotic resistance?

      a. Ampicillin

      b. Gentamicin

      c. Vancomycin

      d. Amoxicillin

16-4. Risk factors for the development of *Clostridium difficile*–associated disease include:

      a. Antibiotic use

      b. Age less than 65 years

      c. Underlying bowel disease

      d. Drinking unfiltered water

16-5. Which of the following are acceptable strategies to prevent antimicrobial resistance in health care settings?

      a. Increase the use of indwelling catheters.

      b. Treat colonization (i.e., tracheal aspirate, bacterial contamination of catheter tip, etc.) to prevent further development of disease.

      c. Use broad spectrum antibiotics.

      d. Vaccinate high-risk patients against influenza.

When penicillin was discovered by Alexander Fleming in the 1920s, scientists rejoiced because a treatment for infections was found. As a result, diseases such as tuberculosis, staphylococcal sepsis, syphilis, gonorrhea, and strep throat were successfully overcome by antibiotics, and millions of lives were saved. Unfortunately, within a few years after penicillin started being routinely used, the first cases of antibiotic resistance were seen. The first bacteria to show resistance to penicillin was *Staphylococcus aureus*. Although *S. aureus* is normally considered an innocuous inhabitant of our skin flora, it can produce disease. In 1967, another type of penicillin-resistant pneumonia caused by *Streptococcus pneumoniae* was found. At about the same time, U.S. military personnel in Southeast Asia were acquiring penicillin-resistant gonorrhea from prostitutes. By 1976, when the soldiers had come home, they brought with them the new strain of gonorrhea that was resistant to penicillin. In 1983, a hospital-acquired intestinal infection caused by the bacterium *Enterococcus faecium* joined the list of bugs that could outwit penicillin.

Antimicrobial resistance occurs when bacteria change or adapt in a way that allows them to survive in the presence of antibiotics designed to kill them. In some cases, microorganisms, predominantly bacteria, become resistant to one or more classes of antimicrobial agents; these multidrug-resistant organisms (MDROs) may be difficult to eradicate because no available antibiotics are effective against them. For example, penicillin kills bacteria by attaching to their cell walls, then destroying a key part of the wall. The wall falls apart and the bacterium dies. Resistant microbes, however, either change their cell walls so penicillin cannot bind, or they produce enzymes that destroy the antibiotic. In another example, erythromycin attacks structures within a bacterial cell that enable it to make proteins (ribosomes). Resistant bacteria have slightly altered ribosomes that do not allow drug binding.

Additionally, all types of bacteria have variants with unusual traits. For example, some bacteria within a species do not die in the presence of a certain antibiotic. When a person takes an antibiotic, the drug kills the susceptible bacteria, leaving behind—or "selecting"—those that can resist it. These resistant bacteria then multiply, increasing their numbers by up to a million-fold a day, becoming the predominant microorganism.

A patient can develop a drug-resistant infection either by contracting a resistant bug or by developing bacterial resistance in the body following antibiotic treatment. MDROs increase a patient's risk of death and are often associated with medical complications and prolonged hospital stays. These might necessitate removing part of an infected lung or colon, removing an intravenous catheter, or replacing a damaged heart valve.

HOW ANTIBIOTIC RESISTANCE HAPPENS

Bacteria can acquire antibiotic resistance in one of three ways: spontaneous DNA mutation, transformation, or plasmid mediated.

In *spontaneous DNA mutation,* the genetic material of the bacteria can change spontaneously to become more drug-resistant. Drug-resistant tuberculosis happens this way.

In *transformation,* bacteria take up DNA from another bacterium through their cell wall that contains genetic material that is resistant to antibiotics. Penicillin-resistant gonorrhea is a result of transformation.

Another way that bacteria develop antibiotic resistance is through *plasmids,* which are small circles of DNA that can carry genes for antibiotic resistance. These plasmids can be transferred from one type of bacterium to another.

These events then cause changes in the bacteria, such as:

- The production of enzymes by the bacteria that degrades or chemically modifies and therefore inactivates the antibiotics. For example, enzymatic deactivation of *Penicillin* G in some penicillin-resistant bacteria through the production of the enzyme, β-lactamase.
- Modification or replacement of molecules or target site on the bacteria that are normally bound by an antibiotic, so there is no target for the antibiotic to bind. For example, alteration of penicillin-binding protein or the binding target site of penicillins—in MRSA and other penicillin-resistant bacteria.
- Alteration of metabolic pathway to improve the survival of the bacteria. For example, sulfonamides work by inhibiting the synthesis of folic acid and other nucleic acids, which are nutrients that bacteria require to survive. Resistant bacteria adapt the ability to use preformed folic acid from the host, just like mammalian cells.
- Decreasing the permeability of a bacterial cell to the antibiotic or the development of efficient efflux pumps to pump out the antibiotic from the bacterial cell before it has reached its target.

PREVENTING ANTIBIOTIC RESISTANCE

Many factors contribute to the emergence and spread of antibiotic resistance (Table 16.1). Although antibiotic resistance is inevitable, there are measures to control the spread of antibiotic resistance. Two of the most important measures are infection control activities (see Chapter 1) and judicious use of antibiotics.

Not all infections require treatment with antibiotics. Many cases of pharyngitis, otitis media, sinusitis, and bronchitis are usually caused by viruses and will not be helped by antibiotics. Antibiotic drugs attack bacteria, not viruses. In addition, the practice of giving antibiotics to prevent ear infections and the use of antibiotic prophylaxis before surgery should conform to evidence-based guidelines. Antibiotics should be restricted to patients who have bacterial infections.

If an antibiotic is necessary, select the most appropriate antibiotic. While using a broad-spectrum antibiotic (one that kills a wide variety of bacteria) may seem logical, this practice actually contributes to the spread of antibiotic resistance. When antibiotics are necessary, an agent that is effective against the most common bacteria for that type of infection should be used. For example, bacterial pharyngitis or sore throat is usually caused by the gram positive organism Group A streptococcus. Consequently, an antibiotic that is effective mainly against this organism should be used. If cultures are taken, the choice of antibiotic should be adjusted based on the bacterial sensitivity profile. Although the use of a broad-spectrum antibiotic may effectively treat pharyngitis caused by Group A streptococcus, this practice could lead to bacterial resistance to the broad-spectrum antibiotic.

In patients in whom an antibiotic is necessary, compliance with the regimen should be stressed. Patients often stop taking the drug too soon because symptoms improve. However, this merely encourages resistant microbes to proliferate. The infection returns a few weeks later, and this time a different drug must be used to treat it.

TABLE **16.1**

Factors Contributing to Antibiotic Resistance

▤ Insufficient surveillance and containment of infections
▤ Nonadherence to appropriate hand hygiene practice
▤ Increasing number of immunocompromised patients
▤ Inadequate decontamination of medical devices and equipment
▤ Lack of antibiotic susceptibility testing
▤ Insufficient isolation and/or cohorting of infected patients
▤ Inappropriate use of antibiotics
▤ Failure to complete antibiotic regimens
▤ Lack of education and training of health care professionals

METHICILLIN-RESISTANT *STAPHYLOCOCCUS AUREUS*

Methicillin-resistant *Staphylococcus aureus* (MRSA) is a type of bacteria that is resistant to certain antibiotics called beta-lactams. Beta-lactam antibiotics include methicillin and other more common antibiotics such as oxacillin, penicillin, and amoxicillin. MRSA is becoming more common in health care settings. According to the Centers for Disease Control and Prevention (CDC) data, the proportion of infections that are antimicrobial resistant has been growing. In 1974, MRSA infections accounted for 2% of the total number of staphylococcus infections; this figure rose to 22% in 1995 and to 63% in 2004 (Klevens et al., 2006). This is concerning because patients infected with MRSA are more likely to have longer, more expensive hospital stays and may be more likely to die as a result of the infection. In 2005 almost 95,000 people developed serious, invasive infections with MRSA, and more than 18,000 persons died during a hospital stay related to these serious MRSA infections.

MRSA occurs most frequently in patients who undergo invasive medical procedures or who have weakened immune systems and are being treated in hospitals and health care facilities such as nursing homes and dialysis centers. MRSA in health care settings commonly causes serious and potentially life-threatening infections, such as bloodstream infections, surgical site infections, or pneumonia.

More recently, community-acquired MRSA (CA-MRSA) is being diagnosed. CA-MRSA is defined as those acquired by otherwise healthy persons who have not been hospitalized in the past year or had a medical procedure (such as dialysis, surgery, catheters). Clusters of CA-MRSA infections have been seen in athletes, military recruits, children, Pacific Islanders, Alaskan Natives, Native Americans, men who have sex with men, and prisoners. CA-MRSA most often presents as skin or soft tissue infection such as a boil or abscess. Patients frequently recall a "spider bite." The involved site is red, swollen, and painful and may have pus or other drainage (Figure 16.1).

MRSA is most commonly spread by someone who is already infected or through someone who is colonized with the bacteria. An individual who is

FIGURE 16.1
MRSA wound infection

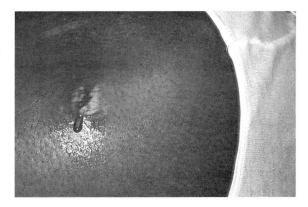

Courtesy of the Centers for Disease Control and Prevention / Bruno Coignard, MD, Jeff Hageman, MHS

colonized carries the bacteria on their bodies but does not have clinical symptoms. While 25% to 30% of the population is colonized with staphylococcus, approximately 1% is colonized with MRSA. The main mode of transmission to other patients is through human hands, especially those of health care workers (HCWs). Hands may become contaminated with MRSA bacteria by contact with infected or colonized patients. If appropriate hand hygiene (see Chapter 1, "Basic Infection Control"), such as washing with soap and water or using an alcohol-based hand sanitizer, is not performed, the bacteria can be spread when the HCW touches other patients. Other factors contributing to transmission include skin-to-skin contact, neckties and other clothing, crowded conditions, and poor hygiene.

In order to diagnose an infection caused by MRSA, a culture should be obtained from the infection site and sent to the microbiology laboratory. For example, in a wound infection, a small biopsy or drainage from the site should be obtained. In patients with suspected pneumonia, a sputum sample should be collected and sent to the microbiology lab. If infection is suspected in the blood or urine, the appropriate specimen should be collected. In the laboratory, if *S. aureus* is isolated, the organism should be tested to determine which antibiotics will be effective for treating the infection.

Technique for Collecting a Wound Culture

- Clean surrounding skin with an antiseptic agent.
- Remove pus, debris, or necrotic tissue from the wound using sterile water or saline.
- Use a sterile syringe to aspirate fresh pus or drainage deep within the wound.
- If aspiration is not possible, insert a sterile swab deep within the wound.

MRSA is preventable. The first step to prevent MRSA is to prevent health care infections in general. Standard infection control precautions should be used for all patients in outpatient and inpatient health care settings. This includes performing hand hygiene after touching body fluids or contaminated items (whether or not gloves are worn), between patients, and when moving from a contaminated body site to a clean site on the same patient; wearing gloves when managing wounds; and wearing gowns and eye protection as appropriate for procedures that are likely to generate splashes or sprays of body fluids. In addition, contact precautions, which involve greater spatial separation of patients (through placing infected patients in private rooms or cohorting patients with similar infection status), use of gown and gloves for all contact with the patient or their environment and use of dedicated noncritical patient-care equipment have been recommended for empiric use in patients with abscesses or draining wounds in which wound drainage cannot be contained. Contact precautions have also been recommended for patients in acute care inpatient settings known or suspected to be infected or colonized with MRSA; these precautions may be modified as appropriate for ambulatory care and other non–acute care inpatient settings based on risk factors for transmission. Exam room surfaces should be cleaned with an EPA-registered hospital detergent/disinfectant, in accordance with label instructions, or a 1:100 solution of diluted bleach (1 tablespoon bleach in 1 quart water).

Several antimicrobial agents have been proposed as alternatives to beta-lactams in the outpatient treatment of skin and soft-tissue infections when an oral regimen with activity against CA-MRSA is needed. These include clindamycin, tetracyclines (including doxycycline and minocycline), trimethoprim-sulfamethoxazole (TMP-SMX), rifampin (used only in combination with other agents), and linezolid. There are advantages and disadvantages to each of these agents. Because of a relatively high prevalence of resistance among *S. aureus* isolates in the community or the potential for rapid development of resistance, some antimicrobial agents are not optimal choices for the empiric treatment of community-associated skin and soft tissue infections possibly caused by *S. aureus*. These include fluoroquinolones and macrolides. More data are needed from controlled clinical trials to establish optimal regimens for the treatment of CA-MRSA.

For treatment of infections caused by MRSA in an inpatient setting, vancomycin is the agent of choice. Alternatives include daptomycin and linezolid, but at the current time, these agents should be reserved for cases that are resistant to vancomycin.

VANCOMYCIN-RESISTANT ENTEROCOCCUS

Enterococci are gram-positive bacteria that are normally present in the human intestines, in the female genital tract, and the in environment. While enterococci can cause infection, in the past, these infections were readily treated with vancomycin. However, vancomycin-resistant enterococci (VRE) were first reported in England and France in 1987 and spread to the United States by 1989. Just 2 years later, 38 hospitals in the United States reported VRE. By 1993, 14% of patients with enterococcal infections in intensive-care units in some hospitals had vancomycin-resistant strains, a 20-fold increase from 1987. The CDC estimates that during 2006 and 2007, about 12% of infections that occurred in the hospital were due to enterococci (CDC, 2008b; Sunenshine & McDonald, 2006). Of these enterococcal infections, about 30% were caused by VRE. In the last decade enterococci have become recognized as a leading cause of health care–associated infections such as bacterial surgical wound and urinary tract infections.

There are a number of risk factors associated with the development of infections with VRE (Table 16.2). VRE is most commonly transmitted person to person by the hands of caregivers. As with MRSA, hands may become contaminated with VRE by contact with a colonized or infected individual or a contaminated surface. VRE can also be spread directly to people after they touch surfaces that are contaminated with VRE. VRE is not usually spread through the air by coughing or sneezing.

The spread of VRE can be contained by following infection control practices. Caregivers should wash hands thoroughly after using the bathroom and

TABLE 16.2

Risk Factors for the Development of VRE Infections

- Long-term treatment with vancomycin or other antibiotics
- Immunocompromised state such as seen in oncology or transplant patients
- Recently surgical procedures such as abdominal or chest surgery
- Prolonged use of indwelling medical devices such as urinary catheters or central intravenous (IV) catheters
- Colonization with VRE

after contact with patients (Figure 16.2). Hands should be washed with soap and water or alcohol-based hand rubs. In addition, judicious use of antibiotics is warranted. For example, use of vancomycin, third-generation cephalosporins, and anti-anaerobic drugs should only be used when indicated by culture and sensitivity reports.

Treatment for VRE colonization is not recommended. However, an aggressive regimen using multiple antibiotics is needed to treat VRE infections. These regimens are selected based on culture and sensitivity information reported by the microbiology laboratory. While some strains of enterococcus can be successfully treated with penicillins such as ampicillin, ampicillin-sulbactam, or penicillin, or vancomycin in combination with an aminoglycoside such as gentamicin or streptomycin, there are strains that are multidrug-resistant and may need antibiotics such as linezolid, daptomycin, tigecycline, or quinupristin-dalfopristin for adequate therapy.

FIGURE 16.2

Appropriate hand washing technique

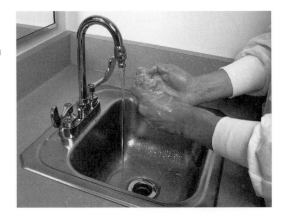

Courtesy of the Centers for Disease Control and Prevention / Kimberly Smith and Christine Ford. Photo by Kimberly Smith.

CLOSTRIDIUM DIFFICILE–ASSOCIATED INFECTIONS

Clostridium difficile is a gram-positive, spore-forming anaerobic bacillus that was first linked to pseudomembranous colitis in 1978. *C. difficile* has been associated with gastrointestinal infections ranging in severity from asymptomatic colonization to severe diarrhea, pseudomembranous colitis, toxic megacolon, intestinal perforation, and death. The incidence and severity of infections caused by *C. difficile* are increasing. Recent reports indicate that a more virulent and possibly more resistant strain of *C. difficile* may be responsible for recent epidemics of *C. difficile*–associated disease (CDAD).

C. difficile toxins can be found in the stool of 15% to 25% of patients with antibiotic-associated diarrhea and more than 95% of patients with pseudomembranous colitis. In U.S. hospitals participating in the National Nosocomial Infections Surveillance System, there were an average of 12.2 reported cases of CDAD per 10,000 patient days in the years 1987 to 1998. Rates were significantly higher in teaching than in nonteaching hospitals (13.0 vs. 11.7 cases per 10,000 patient days), in medical than in surgical services, and in winter months compared with nonwinter months.

Data from the CDC reveal that hospitalizations with a discharge diagnosis of CDAD have almost doubled from 31 per 100,000 patents in 1996 to 61 per 100,000 in 2003. Of patients who contracted *C. difficile* in hospitals or nursing homes, 0.6% to 1.5% died, and CDAD was either the direct or indirect cause of death. Moreover, one study suggests that the severity of observed disease may also be increasing, with a 1-year mortality rate approaching 17% (CDC, 2008a).

There are a variety of risk factors associated with CDAD (Table 16.3). Patients who are hospitalized or those residing in long-term care facilities seem to be at highest risk. The vast majority of *C. difficile* infections occur during or after antimicrobial therapy. Historically, *C. difficile* diarrhea was associated with the use of clindamycin therapy. More recently, almost all antimicrobial agents except for aminoglycosides have been associated with CDAD, and it is thought that

TABLE 16.3

Risk factors for the Development of C. Difficile–*Associated Disease (CDAD)*

- Prolonged hospitalization
- Resident of a long-term care facility
- Treatment with antimicrobial therapy, especially prolonged use of multiple drugs
- Age greater than 65 years
- Severe underlying illness
- Nasogastric intubation
- Antiulcer medications (conflicting evidence)

broad-spectrum antimicrobial agents, which have a greater effect on the normal intestinal flora, are more likely to lead to CDAD. Other studies found fluoroquinolones to be more strongly linked to CDAD than any other antimicrobial agents, including clindamycin and combination beta-lactam/beta-lactamase inhibitors. The risk is also greater when patients receive multiple antimicrobial agents and undergo a longer course of therapy.

As with many other infections, control and prevention of CDAD involves strict adherence to infection control practices. Hand washing is of utmost importance. In addition, patients who are infected with *C. difficile* should be isolated to prevent spread to other individuals.

Treatment of CDAD varies depending on severity of disease. In patients with mild to moderate disease, oral metronidazole remains the mainstay of therapy. In those with more severe disease, oral vancomycin can be considered. In severe, complicated cases, surgery may be warranted. There are a variety of investigational agents for the treatment of *C. difficile,* including tolevamer, ramoplanin, nitazoxanide, rifaximin, and others.

SUMMARY

In summary, infections caused by MDROs are on the rise. There are a number of steps that can help to reduce the spread of these infections. The CDC (2001) recommends the 12 steps in Table 16.4 to prevent antimicrobial resistance in the health care setting.

TABLE 16.4

12 Steps to Prevent Antimicrobial Resistance

PREVENT INFECTION
Step 1: Vaccinate
▣ Give influenza/pneumococcal vaccine to at-risk patients before discharge.
▣ Get influenza vaccine annually.
Step 2: Get the Catheters out
▣ Use catheters only when essential.
▣ Use catheters only when essential.
▣ Use the correct catheter.
▣ Use proper insertion and catheter-care protocols.
▣ Remove catheters when they are no longer essential.

(Continued)

TABLE 16.4

(*Continued*)

DIAGNOSE AND TREAT INFECTION EFFECTIVELY

Step 3: Target the Pathogen

- Culture the patient.
- Target empiric therapy to likely pathogens using local antibiotic resistance information.
- Target definitive therapy to known pathogens and antimicrobial susceptibility test results.

Step 4: Access the Experts

- Consult infectious diseases experts for patients with serious infections.

USE ANTIMICROBIALS WISELY

Step 5: Practice Antimicrobial Control

- Engage in local antimicrobial control efforts.

Step 6: Use Local Data

- Know your antibiogram.
- Know your patient population.

Step 7: Treat Infection, Not Contamination

- Use proper antisepsis for blood and other cultures.
- Culture the blood, not the skin or catheter hub.
- Use proper methods to obtain and process all cultures.

Step 8: Treat infection, Not Colonization

- Treat pneumonia, not the tracheal aspirate.
- Treat bacteremia, not the catheter tip or hub.
- Treat urinary tract infection, not the indwelling catheter.

Step 9: Know When to Say "No" to Vancomycin

- Treat infection, not contaminants or colonization.
- Fever in a patient with an intravenous catheter is not a routine indication for vancomycin.

Step 10: Stop Antimicrobial Treatment:

- When infection is cured.
- When cultures are negative and infection is unlikely.
- When infection is not diagnosed.

PREVENT TRANSMISSION

Step 11: Isolate the Pathogen

- Use standard infection control precautions.

(*Continued*)

TABLE 16.4

(*Continued*)

> ▪ Contain infectious body fluids. (Follow airborne, droplet, and contact precautions.)
>
> ▪ When in doubt, consult infection control experts.
>
> *Step 12: Break the Chain of Contagion*
>
> ▪ Stay home when you are sick.
>
> ▪ Keep your hands clean.
>
> ▪ Set an example.

From the Centers for Disease Control and Prevention (2001).

POST-TEST QUESTIONS

16-1. Which of the following bacteria are associated with antibiotic resistance?
   a. *Staphylococcus aureus*
   b. Enterococci
   c. *Clostridium difficile*
   d. All of the above

16-2. One of the most important measures of control of antibiotic resistance is:
   a. Judicious use of antibiotics
   b. Hepatitis C infections
   c. Increasing number of viral infections
   d. All of the above

16-3. Overuse of which of the following antibiotics has been associated with antibiotic resistance?
   a. Ampicillin
   b. Gentamicin
   c. Vancomycin
   d. Amoxicillin

16-4. Risk factors for the development of Clostridium difficile–associated disease include:
   a. Antibiotic use
   b. Age less than 65 years
   c. Underlying bowel disease
   d. Drinking unfiltered water

16-5. Which of the following are acceptable strategies to prevent antimicrobial resistance in healthcare settings?
   a. Increase the use of indwelling catheters.
   b. Treat colonization (i.e., tracheal aspirate, bacterial contamination of catheter tip, etc.) to prevent further development of disease.
   c. Use broad spectrum antibiotics.
   d. Vaccinate high-risk patients against influenza.

References

Centers for Disease Control and Prevention. (2001). *Campaign to prevent antimicrobial resistance in healthcare settings.* Retrieved January 25, 2009, from http://www.cdc.gov/drugresistance/healthcare/identitypiece.htm

Centers for Disease Control and Prevention. (2002). Guidelines for hand hygiene in healthcare settings. Recommendations of the healthcare infection control practices advisory committee and the HICPAC/SHEA/APIC/IDSA hand hygiene task force. *MMWR, 51*(RR-16), 1–45.

Centers for Disease Control and Prevention. (2007). *Healthcare-associated methicillin resistant Staphylococcus aureus (HA-MRSA).* Retrieved January 25, 2009, from http://www.cdc.gov/ncidod/dhqp/ar_mrsa.html

Centers for Disease Control and Prevention. (2008a). *Clostridium difficile infections.* Retrieved January 25, 2009, from http://www.cdc.gov/ncidod/dhqp/id_Cdiff.html

Centers for Disease Control and Prevention. (2008b). *Vancomycin-resistant enterococci (VRE).* Retrieved January 25, 2009, from http://www.cdc.gov/ncidod/dhqp/ar_vre.html

Centers for Disease Control and Prevention. (2009). *Get Smart: Know when antibiotics work.* Retrieved January 25, 2009, from http://www.cdc.gov/getsmart

Klevens, R. M., Edwards, J. R., Tenover, F. C., McDonald, L. C., Horan, T., Gaynes, R., et al. (2006). Changes in the epidemiology of methicillin-resistant *Staphylococcus aureus* in intensive care units in US hospitals, 1992-2003. *Clinical Infectious Disease, 42*(3), 389-391.

Sunenshine, R. H., & McDonald, L. C. (2006). *Clostridium difficile*-associated disease: New challenges from an established pathogen. *Cleveland Clinic Journal of Medicine, 73,* 187-197.

Bioterrorism

17

This chapter includes topics on botulism and smallpox infection. The categorical classification of bioterrorism agents is reviewed. The content differentiates between the chicken pox rash and the smallpox rash. There is discussion on smallpox vaccination site reaction. Finally, the plague and anthrax are discussed.

OBJECTIVES

1. List the signs and symptoms of botulism infection.
2. Identify the steps for smallpox vaccination.
3. Distinguish between the rashes seen with chickenpox versus the rash seen with smallpox.
4. List the types of precautions necessary when caring for a patient with plague.
5. Identify two antibiotics commonly used in the treatment of anthrax disease.

PRE-TEST QUESTIONS

17-1. Symptoms of botulism usually include:
   a. Fever
   b. Mental confusion
   c. Difficulty swallowing
   d. Blister-like rash

17-2. The rash seen in chicken pox:
   a. Is vesicular with a depressed center
   b. Crusts all at the same time
   c. Appears primarily on the trunk
   d. Indicates you are no longer infectious (once the rash appears)

17-3. The rash seen in small pox:
   a. Is flat and red
   b. Usually leaves permanent scars
   c. Indicates that you will not survive
   d. Appears in crops of different stages

17-4. Patients infected with naturally occurring anthrax require:
   a. Standard precautions
   b. Droplet precautions
   c. Airborne precautions
   d. Contact precautions
17-5. Which of the following is a true statement about plague?
   a. Buboes are seen in all forms of plague.
   b. Plague is transmitted by contact with infected livestock and dairy products.
   c. Rodent and rodent fleas carry *Yersina pestis*.
   d. Patients infected with pneumonic plague require airborne precautions.

Bioterrorism is the deliberate release of viruses, bacteria, or other germs (agents) used to intentionally cause illness or death in people, animals, or plants. Most often, the agent used for a bioterrorism attack is a naturally occurring substance (e.g., ricin), virus (e.g., viral hemorrhagic fever), or bacteria (e.g. anthrax, plague, smallpox) that has been altered to make it more harmful to its intended target. Biological agents can be spread through the air, through water, or in food. These agents are often difficult to detect initially, and by the time the substance has been detected, it has already spread extensively.

Agents used in bioterrorism are separated into three categories, depending on how easily they can be spread and the severity of illness or death they cause (Centers for Disease Control and Prevention [CDC], 2007). Category A agents are considered the highest risk. Examples of bioterrorism agents that are considered category A include anthrax (*Bacillus anthracis*), botulism (*Clostridium botulinum toxin*), plague (*Yersinia pestis*), smallpox (variola major), tularemia (*Francisella tularensis*), and viral hemorrhagic fevers. Category B agents are considered to be of moderate risk. Examples of category B agents include brucellosis (*Brucella* species), food (e.g., *Salmonella* species, *Escherichia coli* O157:H7, *Shigella*), and water (e.g., *Vibrio cholerae, Cryptosporidium parvum*) threats. Category C agents are those that are considered emerging threats for disease. An example of a category C threat is the hantavirus.

The following are categorical classifications of bioterrorism agents.

Category A

▪ High-priority agents posing the highest risk to the public and national security
▪ Easily spread or transmitted from person to person
▪ Potential for high death rates and for major public health impact
▪ Potential to cause public panic and social disruption
▪ Require special action for public health preparedness

Category B

▪ Second highest priority
▪ Moderately easy to spread

- Result in moderate rates of illness and death
- Require specific enhancements of CDC's laboratory capacity and enhanced disease monitoring

Category C

- Include emerging pathogens that could be engineered for mass spread in the future
- Easily available
- Easily produced and spread
- Potential for high morbidity and mortality rates and major health impact.

This chapter discusses a number of the bioterrorism agents that are considered category A, including anthrax, botulism, plague, and smallpox.

ANTHRAX

Anthrax is caused by the encapsulated, aerobic, gram-positive, spore-forming, rod-shaped (bacillus) bacterium *Bacillus anthracis*. Anthrax can affect three different body systems: the skin (cutaneous anthrax), lungs (inhalation anthrax), or the digestive system (gastrointestinal anthrax). In general, anthrax does not spread from person to person, but rather it is spread by handling products from infected animals (for example, cattle, sheep, goats, camels, antelopes) or by breathing in anthrax spores produced by the bacteria, which can live in the soil for many years or be in infected animal products (e.g., wool). People also can become infected by eating undercooked meat or dairy products from infected animals. Unfortunately, anthrax has also been used as an agent of bioterrorism. In 2001, anthrax was intentionally spread through the postal system by sending letters with powder containing anthrax. This caused more than 20 cases of anthrax infection and a number of anthrax-related deaths.

The symptoms of anthrax vary depending on the body system that is infected. Typically, patients begin to experience symptoms within 7 days of coming in contact with the bacteria or spores, but the onset can be delayed by up to 6 weeks with inhalational anthrax. The most common infection caused by anthrax is cutaneous anthrax. In cutaneous anthrax, patients may notice a papular that turns into a vesicle (see Figure 17.1). Over time, the painless vesicle becomes an ulcer with an eschar. If anthrax is ingested, the most common initial symptoms are nausea, anorexia, bloody diarrhea, and fever, which progress to severe abdominal pains. Within 2 to 4 days after onset of the initial symptoms, patients develop ascites followed by shock and death within 2 to 5 days, if left untreated. Finally, if the spores of the anthrax bacteria are inhaled, patients may initially feel like they have a cold or flu. For example, they may experience sore throat, mild fever, and myalgias, which over time progresses to cough, chest discomfort, dyspnea, and fatigue. Over the next 1 to 5 days the patient can experience an abrupt onset of high fever and severe respiratory distress comprising of dyspnea, stridor, and cyanosis. If left untreated, shock and death can occur within 24–36 hours (Inglesby et al., 2002).

FIGURE **17.1**

Cutaneous anthrax infection

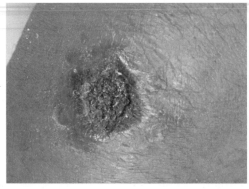

Courtesy of the Centers for Disease Control and Prevention / James H. Steele.

Once anthrax infection is suspected or diagnosed, patients are started on antibiotics. Examples of antibiotics that have successfully been used in the treatment of anthrax infections include ciprofloxacin, levofloxacin, doxycycline, and penicillins such as amoxicillin. Treatment should be continued for 60 days.

Standard precautions should be used for all types of anthrax. Standard precautions should include the routine use of gloves for contact with nonintact skin, including rashes and skin lesions. Patients do not have to be maintained in a private room because anthrax is not transmitted through the airborne route. (Inglesby et al., 2002)

There is a vaccine to prevent anthrax, but it is not yet available for the general public. For now, the vaccine is only for people who are at high risk of being exposed to the bacteria. These groups include certain members of the U.S. armed forces, laboratory workers, and workers who may enter or re-enter contaminated areas. The immunization consists of three subcutaneous injections given 2 weeks apart followed by three additional subcutaneous injections given at 6, 12, and 18 months. Annual booster injections of the vaccine are needed to maintain immunity. In the event of a bioterrorism attack, people exposed would also get the vaccine.

BOTULISM

Clostridium botulinum is an anaerobic gram-positive bacillus that produces a botulinum toxin, which affects the central nervous system. Botulinum toxin inhibits the release of acetylcholine, resulting in characteristic flaccid paralysis often associated with botulism. *C. botulinum* produces spores that are present in soil and marine sediment throughout the world. There are three main forms of botulism: foodborne botulism, which occurs when a person ingests pre-formed toxin that leads to illness within a few hours to days; infant botulism, which occurs in a small number of susceptible infants each year who ingest *C. botulinum,* which produces toxin in the intestinal tract; and wound botulism, which occurs when wounds are infected with *C. botulinum* that secretes the toxin. Foodborne botulism is the most common form of disease in adults. Botulinum toxin is most often transmitted by ingestion of toxin-contaminated food. Botulism is not transmitted from person to person. Aerosolization of botulinum toxin may be a mechanism for a bioterrorism attack resulting in an inhalation form of botulism. However, this form does not occur naturally and is only seen in the case of a bioterrorism attack (Arnon, 2001).

Symptoms of foodborne botulism begin 12–36 hours (but up to 10 days) after ingestion; in the case of inhalational botulism, symptoms begin 24–72 hours after aerosol exposure. Usually patients do not have a fever but will have an intact mental state. Patients with botulism usually experience neurologic symptoms that include double vision, blurred vision, drooping eyelids, slurred speech, difficulty swallowing, dry mouth, and muscle weakness that moves down the body, usually affecting the shoulders first, then the upper arms, lower arms, thighs, calves, and so forth. If respiratory paralysis occurs, patients will die unless mechanical ventilation is provided.

Once botulism infection is suspected or diagnosed, antitoxin should be administered. A supply of antitoxin against infant botulism is maintained by the California Department of Public Health's Infant Botulism Treatment and Prevention Program, and a supply of antitoxin against other kinds of botulism is maintained by the CDC. The antitoxin is most effective in reducing the severity of symptoms if administered early in the course of the disease. Most patients eventually recover after weeks to months of supportive care (Arnon, 2001).

Standard precautions should be used for all types of botulism. Patients do not have to be maintained in a private room because botulism is not transmitted through the airborne route. Contaminated objects or surfaces should be cleaned with 0.1% hypochlorite bleach solution if they cannot be avoided for the hours to days required for natural degradation.

Heating to an internal temperature of 85°C for at least 5 minutes will detoxify contaminated food or drink. In the case of potential inhalational exposure, some protection may be conferred by covering the mouth and nose with clothing. Intact skin is impermeable to botulinum toxin and is not a mode of transmission. A pentavalent toxoid vaccine has been developed by the Department of Defense. However, this vaccine is only available as an investigational new drug and is not commercially available. Patients who require the vaccine typically receive a three-dose series (0, 2, 12 weeks). Routine immunization of the public, including health care workers, is not currently recommended (Arnon, 2001).

PLAGUE

Plague is a disease caused by the gram-negative bacillus bacterium *Yersinia pestis* (*Y. pestis*), which is found in rodents and rodent fleas worldwide. Each year, there are 1,000 to 3,000 cases of naturally occurring cases of plague. There are two forms of the plague: bubonic and pneumonic. Most cases of plague are the bubonic form of the disease. Bubonic plague is transmitted through the bite of an infected flea or exposure to *Y. pestis* through a break in the skin; it cannot be transmitted from person to person. However, if bubonic plague is not treated, the bacteria can spread through the bloodstream and infect the lungs, causing a secondary case of pneumonic plague. Naturally occurring pneumonic plague is uncommon, although small outbreaks do occur. Pneumonic plague affects the lungs and is transmitted when a person breathes in respiratory droplets of *Y. pestis* particles in the air. Respiratory droplets are spread most readily by coughing or sneezing. A bioweapon carrying *Y. pestis* is possible because *Y. pestis* occurs naturally and can be grown in large quantities in a laboratory. If used in an aerosol attack, *Y. pestis* could cause cases of the pneumonic form of plague (Inglesby et al., 2000).

Symptoms of bubonic plague include swollen, tender lymph glands called buboes. Buboes do not occur in pneumonic plague. Patients with bubonic plague may also experience fever, headache, chills, and weakness. In pneumonic plague, symptoms develop 1 to 6 days after becoming infected with the bacteria and include fever, weakness, and rapidly developing pneumonia with dyspnea, chest pain, cough, and sometimes bloody or watery sputum. Nausea, vomiting, and abdominal pain may also occur. Without early treatment, pneumonic plague usually leads to respiratory failure, shock, and rapid death (Inglesby et al., 2000).

Antibiotic treatment is the mainstay of therapy for bubonic and pneumonic plague. People who have had close contact with an infected person should begin a 7-day course of prophylactic antibiotics within 7 days, preferably within 24 hours, of exposure. Infected patients should be treated with antibiotics taken for at least 7 days. Antibiotics that have been used to treat and prevent plague include doxycycline and ciprofloxacin. Alternatives include the intravenous use of cloramphenicol, streptomycin, or gentamicin (Inglesby et al., 2000).

Yersinia pestis is easily destroyed by sunlight and drying. Even so, when released into air, the bacterium will survive for up to 1 hour, depending on conditions. For bubonic plague, standard precautions are necessary. For pneumonic plague, droplet precautions should be used in addition to standard precautions. Persons in contact with a patient with pneumonic plague should wear a surgical-type mask. Droplet precautions should be maintained until the patient has completed 72 hours of antimicrobial therapy. Because of the potential for droplet transmission, patients with suspected or diagnosed pneumonic plague should be maintained in a private room, or patients with similar symptoms and the same presumptive diagnosis (i.e., pneumonic plague) should be cohorted when private rooms are not available (Inglesby et al., 2000).

Currently, plague vaccine is not available in the United States.

SMALLPOX

Smallpox is caused by the orthopox virus, variola virus. Humans are the only natural hosts of variola. Smallpox has been described in humans for thousands of years but has been eradicated from the world. The last natural outbreak of smallpox in the United States occurred in 1949, and by 1972 routine smallpox vaccinations for children in the United States were no longer required. However, there are stockpiles of the virus in laboratories. As a result, there is heightened concern that the variola virus might be used as an agent of bioterrorism. Smallpox is a serious, contagious, and potentially fatal disease. There are two clinical forms of smallpox. Variola major is the severe and most common form of smallpox, with a more extensive rash and higher fever. Variola minor is a less common presentation of smallpox and a much less severe disease. Transmission of smallpox occurs after direct and prolonged person-to-person contact. Smallpox also can be spread through direct contact with infected bodily fluids or contaminated objects such as bedding or clothing. Rarely, smallpox has been spread by virus carried in the air in enclosed settings such as buildings, buses, and trains. A person with smallpox is sometimes contagious with onset of fever but becomes most contagious with the onset of rash (first 7 to 10 days). They remain contagious until the last smallpox scab falls off (Henderson et al., 1999).

The initial symptoms of smallpox or the prodrome include fever, malaise, head and body aches, and sometimes vomiting. The fever is usually high, in the range of 101 to 104 degrees Fahrenheit. This phase typically lasts for 2 to 4 days. Approximately 4 days after the onset of the prodrome, a rash emerges as small red spots on the tongue and in the mouth. These spots develop into sores that break open and spread large amounts of the virus into the mouth and throat. Around the time the sores in the mouth break down, a rash appears on the skin, starting on the face and spreading to the arms and legs and then to the hands and feet. Usually the rash spreads to all parts of the body within 24 hours. As the rash appears, the fever usually improves. By the third day of the rash, the rash becomes raised bumps. By the fourth day, the bumps become pustules and fill with a thick, opaque fluid and often have a depression in the center (see Figure 17.2). Fever may rise again at this time and remain high until scabs form over the bumps. Around the fifth day, the pustules begin to form a crust and then scab. Most of the sores have scabbed over about 2 weeks after the rash appears. Unlike the rash of varicella (chicken pox), where the pox occur in crops, a smallpox rash has a synchronous onset and occurs predominantly on the extremities (see Figure 17.3). The majority of patients with smallpox recover, but in up to 30% of cases, the disease is fatal. Many smallpox survivors have permanent scars over large areas of their body and face (Henderson et al., 1999).

FIGURE 17.2

Typical smallpox rash

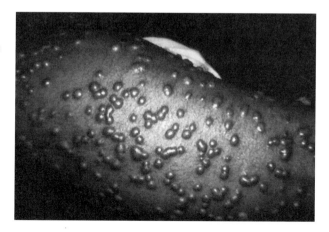

Courtesy of the Centers for Disease Control and Prevention / John Noble, Jr.

FIGURE **17.3**

Difference between
distribution of smallpox
and chickenpox rash

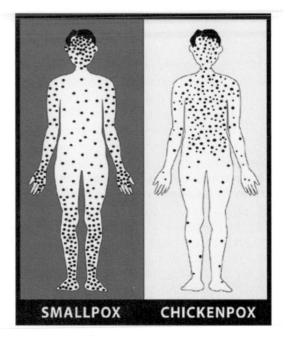

Courtesy of the Centers for Disease Control and Prevention.

There is no proven treatment for smallpox, but research to evaluate the antiviral agent cidofovir, as well as a vaccinia immune globulin, is underway. Supportive therapy is administered (e.g., intravenous fluids, antipyretics, and analgesics) along with antibiotics for any secondary bacterial infections that may occur. Patients who had smallpox and survived are immune to the disease.

As with any unidentified rash illness, patients with suspected smallpox should be isolated in a negative air pressure room. Airborne and contact precautions should be used in addition to standard precautions. Anyone caring for a smallpox patient should wear a NIOSH-approved N95 mask. Caregivers and visitors should wear clean gloves upon entry into the patient room and a gown for all patient contact and for all contact with the patient's environment. The gown must be removed prior to leaving the patient's room. Hands should be washed using an antimicrobial agent (Siegel, Rhinehart, Jackson, Chiarello, & the Healthcare Infection Control Practices Advisory Committee [HICPAC], 2007). Patient placement in a private room is preferred, however, in the event of a large outbreak; patients who have active infections with the same disease may be cohorted in rooms that meet appropriate ventilation and airflow requirements for airborne precautions (Henderson et al., 1999).

Prevention of smallpox can be achieved through vaccination. If a person is vaccinated before exposure to smallpox, the vaccine can completely protect them. Vaccination within 3 days after exposure will prevent or greatly lessen the severity of smallpox in most people. Vaccination 4 to 7 days after exposure likely offers some protection from disease or may decrease the severity of

TABLE 17.1

Technique for Administering the Smallpox Vaccine

■ *Dip needle.* The needle is dipped into the vaccine vial and withdrawn. The needle is designed to hold a tiny drop of vaccine of sufficient size and strength to ensure a take if properly administered. The same needle should never be dipped into the vaccine vial more than once (Figure 17.5).

■ *Make perpendicular insertions within a 5-mm diameter area.* The needle is held perpendicular to the site of insertion. The wrist of the vaccinator should be maintained in a firm position by resting on the arm of the vaccinee or another firm support (Figure 17.6).

■ *A number of perpendicular insertions are made in rapid order in an area approximately 5 mm in diameter.* The number of insertions should be in accordance with the package insert, using 15 insertions for all vaccinees. A trace of blood should appear at the site of vaccination within 15–20 seconds.

■ *The bifurcated needle is for one-time use only and should be discarded in an appropriate biohazard container immediately after vaccinating each patient.*

■ *Absorb excess vaccine.* After vaccination; excess vaccine should be absorbed with sterile gauze. Discard the gauze in a safe manner (usually in an infection control receptacle) in order not to contaminate the site or infect others who may come in contact with it.

■ *Cover vaccination site. I*t is important that the vaccination site be covered to prevent dissemination of virus. Gauze should be loosely secured by first aid adhesive tape (Figure 17.7).

  ● When working in a health care setting, vaccinees should keep their vaccination site covered with gauze or a similar absorbent material. This dressing should, in turn, be covered with a semipermeable dressing. Products combining an absorbent base with an overlying semipermeable layer also can be used to cover the vaccination site. Health care workers do not need to be placed on leave after receiving a smallpox vaccination.

  ● Vaccinees in settings where close personal contact is likely (such as parents of infants and young children) should cover the vaccination site with gauze or a similar absorbent material, wear a shirt or other clothing that would cover the vaccination site, and also make sure to practice good hand hygiene.

From the Centers for Disease Control and Prevention.

disease. Vaccination will not protect smallpox patients who already have a rash. Smallpox vaccination provides immunity for 3 to 5 years and decreases thereafter. Upon repeat vaccination, immunity lasts longer. Historically, the vaccine has been effective in preventing smallpox infection in 95% of those vaccinated. (Henderson et al., 1999)

Vaccination must be performed using a bifurcated or two-pronged needle (Figure 17.4) using a specified technique (Table 17.1). Vaccination is generally in the deltoid area on the upper arm. Alcohol should not be applied to the skin prior to vaccination because alcohol can inactivate the vaccine virus.

FIGURE 17.4

Bifurcated needle

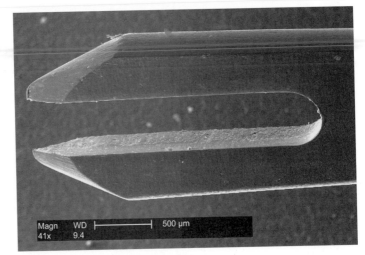

Courtesy of the Centers for Disease Control and Prevention. Photo by Janice Carr.

FIGURE 17.5

Dipping the bifurcated needle into vial

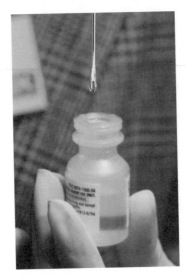

Courtesy of the Centers for Disease Control and Prevention. Photo by James Gathany.

FIGURE 17.6

Making perpendicular insertion into skin

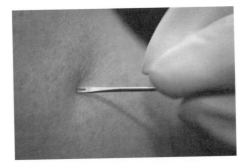

Courtesy of the Centers for Disease Control and Prevention. Photo by James Gathany.

FIGURE 17.7

Example of how to cover smallpox vaccination site

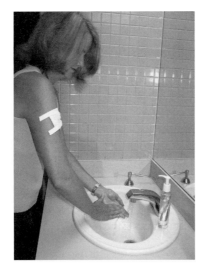

Courtesy of the Centers for Disease Control and Prevention / Kelly Thomas.

To avoid transmission of the virus following vaccination, patients should be instructed to keep the site covered and not touch the area (Table 17.2).

If the vaccination is successful, a red and itchy bump develops at the vaccine site in 3 or 4 days. In the first week, the bump becomes a large blister, fills with pus, and begins to drain. During the second week, the blister begins to dry up and a scab forms. The scab falls off in the third week, leaving a small scar (see Figure 17.8). People who are being vaccinated for the first time have a stronger reaction than those who are being revaccinated (Figure 17.9).

TABLE 17.2

Preventing Transmission of Smallpox after Vaccination

- Do not rub or scratch the vaccination site.

- Keep the site covered and change gauze-only dressings every 1–2 days or if wet. Change semipermeable dressings at least every 3–5 days.

- Keep the vaccination site dry, covering it with a water-proof bandage while bathing.

- Discard gauze carefully in plastic zip bags.

- Set aside a laundry hamper for clothes, towels, sheets, and other items that may come into contact with the vaccination site.

- Wash clothing or other materials that come into contact with the vaccination site in hot water with detergent and/or bleach. Wash hands afterward.

- Wash hands thoroughly with soap and hot water or with alcohol-based hand rubs such as gels or foams after touching the vaccination site, or bandages, clothing, towels, or sheets that have come into contact with the vaccination site.

- When the scab falls off, throw it away in a plastic zip bag.

FIGURE 17.8

The primary smallpox vaccination site reaction

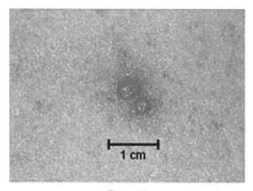

Day 4

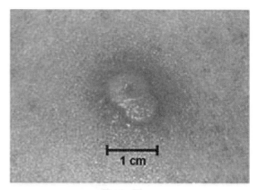

Day 7

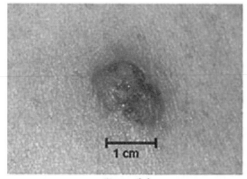

Day 14

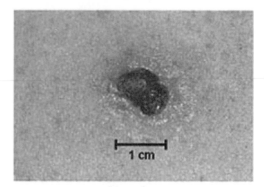

Day 21

Courtesy of the Centers for Disease Control and Prevention.

FIGURE 17.9

Generalized vaccinia
reaction after smallpox
vaccine

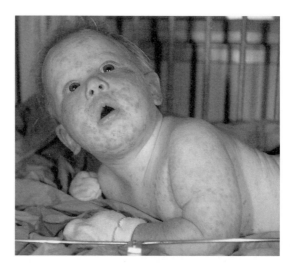

Courtesy of the Centers for Disease Control and Prevention, Allen W. Mathies, MD, California
Emergency Preparedness Office (Calif/EPO). Immunization Branch. Photo by Allen W. Mathies.

For individuals involved in administering smallpox vaccine, a pocket guide is available showing the vaccination method, reactions, and contraindications (CDC, 2003).

ROLE OF THE HEALTH CARE PROFESSIONAL

Hospitals and clinics will likely be the first group to recognize a bioterrorism attack. It is vital that they act quickly and appropriately. Health care facilities should have infection control policies in place to rapidly implement prevention and control measures in response to a suspected outbreak. Should a bioterrorism event be suspected, communication is imperative to limit the spread of the disease. Information must be rapidly communicated to infection control personnel, health care administration, local and state health departments, the Federal Bureau of Investigation (FBI) field office, and the CDC. Existing local emergency plans should be reviewed and a multidisciplinary approach outlined that includes local emergency medical services (EMS), police and fire departments, and media relations in addition to health care providers and IC professionals. Annual disaster-preparedness drills held at many facilities can improve response capacity by incorporating a bioterrorism scenario to test and refine bioterrorism readiness plans at each individual facility (APIC Bioterrorism Task Force and CDC Hospital Infections Program Bioterrorism Working Group, 1999).

POST-TEST QUESTIONS

17-1. Symptoms of botulism usually include:
    a. Fever
    b. Mental confusion
    c. Difficulty swallowing
    d. Blister-like rash

17-2. The rash seen in chicken pox:
    a. Is vesicular with a depressed center
    b. Crusts all at the same time
    c. Appears primarily on the trunk
    d. Indicates you are no longer infectious (once the rash appears)

17-3. The rash seen in small pox:
    a. Is flat and red
    b. Usually leaves permanent scars
    c. Indicates that you will not survive
    d. Appear in crops of different stages

17-4. Patients infected with naturally occurring anthrax require:
    a. Standard precautions
    b. Droplet precautions
    c. Airborne precautions
    d. Contact precautions

17-5. Which of the following is a true statement about plague:

    a. Buboes are seen in all forms of plague.

    b. Plague is transmitted by contact with infected livestock and dairy products.

    c. Rodent and rodent fleas carry *Yersina pestis.*

    d. Patients infected with pneumonic plague require airborne precautions.

References

APIC Bioterrorism Task Force and CDC Hospital Infections Program Bioterrorism Working Group. (1999). *Bioterrorism readiness plan: A template for healthcare facilities.* Retrieved from http://www.cdc.gov/ncidod/dhqp/pdf/bt/13apr99APIC-CDCBioterrorism.PDF

Arnon, S.S., Schechter, R., Inglesby, T.V., et al. (2001). Botulinum toxin as a biological weapon: Medical and public health management. *JAMA, 285*(8), 1059–1070.

Centers for Disease Control and Prevention. (2003). *Smallpox vaccination.* Retrieved from http://emergency.cdc.gov/training/smallpoxvaccine/reactions/SmallpoxVaccinationGuide.pdf

Centers for Disease Control and Prevention. (2007). *Emergency preparedness and response: Bioterrorism overview.* Retrieved from http://emergency.cdc.gov/bioterrorism/overview.asp

Inglesby, T.V., Dennis, D.T., Henderson, D.A., et al. (2000). Plague as a biological weapon: Medical and public health management. *JAMA, 283*(17), 2281–2290.

Inglesby, T.V., O'Toole, T., Henderson, D.A., et al. (2002). Anthrax as a biological weapon, 2002: Updated recommendations for management. *JAMA, 287*(17), 2236–2252.

Henderson, D.A., Inglesby, T.V., Bartlett, J.G., et al. (1999). Smallpox as a biological weapon: Medical and public health management. *JAMA, 281*(22), 2127–2137.

Siegel, J.D., Rhinehart, E., Jackson, M., Chiarello, L., & the Healthcare Infection Control Practices Advisory Committee (HICPAC). (2007). 2007 Guideline for isolation precautions: Preventing transmission of infectious agents in healthcare settings. Retrieved July 14, 2010, from: http://www.cdc.gov/ncidod/dhqp/pdf/isolation2007.pdf

Suggested Reading

General Bioterrorism Infection Control

Recognition of illness associated with the intentional release of a biologic agent. (2001). *MMWR, 50*(41), 893–897.

Anthrax

Centers for Disease Control and Prevention. (n.d.). Anthrax. Retrieved from http://emergency.cdc.gov/agent/anthrax/

Botulism

Centers for Disease Control and Prevention. (n.d.). Botulism. Retrieved from http://emergency.cdc.gov/agent/botulism/

Sobel, J. (2005). Botulism. *Clin Infect Dis, 41*, 1167–1173.

Plague

Centers for Disease Control and Prevention. (n.d.). Plague. Retrieved from http://emergency.cdc.gov/agent/plague/

Smallpox

Centers for Disease Control and Prevention. (n.d.). Smallpox. Retrieved from http://emer gency.cdc.gov/agent/smallpox/

Centers for Disease Control and Prevention. (2003). Recommendations for using smallpox vaccine in a pre-event vaccination program. Supplemental recommendations of the Advisory Committee on Immunization Practices (ACIP) and the Healthcare Infection Control Practices Advisory Committee (HICPAC). *MMWR*, *52*(RR07), 1–16.

Answer Key

Chapter 1

1. C
2. A
3. C
4. B
5. D

Chapter 2

1. C
2. D
3. A
4. A
5. D

Chapter 3

1. D
2. A
3. D
4. C
5. D

Chapter 4

1. A
2. D
3. C
4. B
5. A

Chapter 5

1. D
2. D
3. B
4. B
5. A

Chapter 6

1. E
2. B
3. E
4. E
5. E

Chapter 7

1. A
2. D
3. B
4. A
5. A

Chapter 8

1. A
2. D
3. B
4. B
5. A

Chapter 9

1. A
2. D
3. B
4. C
5. A

Chapter 10

1. C
2. A
3. D
4. A
5. A

Chapter 11

1. A
2. B
3. C
4. B
5. D

Chapter 12

1. C
2. A
3. D
4. A
5. B

Chapter 13

1. D
2. A
3. D
4. B
5. C

Chapter 14

1. A
2. A
3. D
4. D
5. A

Chapter 15

1. B
2. A
3. C
4. C
5. B

Chapter 16

1. D
2. A
3. C
4. A
5. D

Chapter 17

1. C
2. C
3. B
4. A
5. C

Acronyms

AAFP	American Academy of Family Physicians
AAP	American Academy of Pediatrics
ACIP	Advisory Committee on Immunization Practices
AIA	American Institute of Architects
AIDS	Acquired immune deficiency syndrome
APIC	Association for Professionals in Infection Control and Epidemiology
AZT	Azidothymidine (Zidovudine)
BCCDC	British Columbia Centre for Disease Control
BCG	Bacillus Calmette-Guérin
BSI	Bloodstream infection
CA-MRSA	Community-aquired methicillin-resistant *Staphylococcus Aureus*
CAUTI	Catheter-associated urinary tract infection
CCU	Coronary care unit
CDAD	Clostridium difficile–associated disease
CDC	Centers for Disease Control and Prevention
CFU	Colony-forming units
CLIA	Clinical Laboratory Improvement Amendments
CMS	Centers for Medicare and Medicaid Service
CRS	Congenital rubella syndrome
C\S	Cesarean section
CVC	Central venous catheter
DFU	Direction for use
DOH	Department of Health
DOT	Directly observed therapy
DVT	Deep vein thrombosis
EPA	Environmental Protection Agency
ESRD	End-stage renal disease
FDA	Food and Drug Administration
GBS	Group B Streptococcus
HAI	Health care–associated infection

HASMAT	Hazardous materials
HAV	Hepatitis A virus
HbeAg	Hepatitis B e antigen
HbsAg	Hepatitis B surface antigen
HBV	Hepatitis B virus
HCF	Health care facility
HCP	Health care provider
HCV	Hepatitis C virus
HCW	Health care worker
HEPA	High-efficiency particulate air
HICPAC	Health care Infection Control Practices Advisory Committee
HIGB	Hepatitis B immunoglobulin
HIV	Human immunodeficiency virus
HSV	Herpes simplex virus
ICP	Infection control professional
IDLH	Immediately dangerous to life or health
INH	Isoniazid
IPV	Inactivated polio vaccine
IUGR	Intrauterine growth retardation
IUPC	Intrauterine pressure catheter
LAIV	Live attenuated influenza vaccine
LOS	Length of stay
MCV4	Tetravalent meningococcal conjugate vaccine
MDRO	Multidrug-resistant organism
MDR-TB	Multidrug-resistant tuberculosis (MDR-TB)
mg/m3	Milligrams per cubic meter
MMR	Measles mumps rubella
MODS assay	Microscopic-observation drug-susceptibility
MPPCF	Millions of particles per cubic foot of air
MPSV4	Quadrivalent polysaccharide meningococcal vaccine
MRSA	Methicillin-resistant *Staphylococcus aureus*
MSDS	Material safety data sheet
NIOSH	National Institute for Occupational Safety and Health
OP	Outpatient
OPIM	Other potentially infectious material
OPV	Oral poliovirus vaccine
OSHA	Occupational Safety and Health Administration
PAP	Papanicolaou smear

PCV7	7-valent pneumococcal conjugate vaccine
PEL	Permissible exposure limit
PEP	Post-exposure prophylaxis
PHN	Postherpetic neuralgia
PICC	Peripherally inserted central catheter
PICU	Pediatric intensive care unit
PID	Pelvic inflammatory disease
POCT	Point-of-care testing
PPD	Purified protein derivative
PPE	Personal protective equipment
PPI	Proton pump inhibitor
PPM	Parts per million
PPS	Prospective payment system
PPSV23	23-valent pneumococcal polysaccharide vaccine
QFT test	QuantiFERON-TB Gold
REL	Recommended exposure limit
RMW	Regulated medical waste
SARS	Severe acute respiratory syndrome
SPHM	Safe patient handling and movement
SSI	Surgical site infection
STEL	Short-term exposure limit
STI	Sexually transmitted infection
TB	Tuberculosis
TIV	Inactivated influenza vaccine
TJC	The Joint Commission
TMP/SMX	Trimethoprim/sulfamethoxazole
TORCH	Toxoplasma, other, rubella, cytomegalovirus, herpes simplex (*see Glossary definition*)
TST	Tuberculin skin test
TWA	Time weighted average
UTI	Urinary tract infection
VAP	Ventilator-associated pneumonia
VIS	Vaccine information statement
VRE	Vancomycin resistant enterococci
VZIG	Varicella zoster immunoglobulin
VZV	Varicella zoster virus
WHO	World Health Organization
ZDV	Zidovudine

Appendix: Resources

 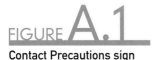
Contact Precautions sign

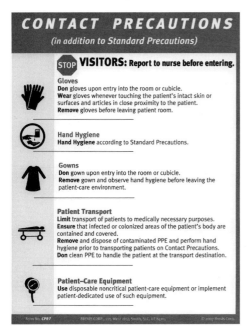

 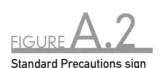
Standard Precautions sign

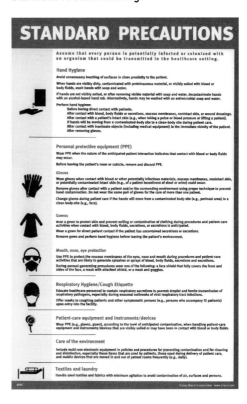

FIGURE **A.3**

Airborne Precautions sign

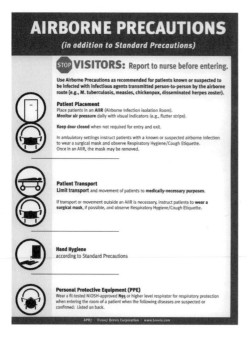

FIGURE **A.4**

Neutropenic Precautions sign

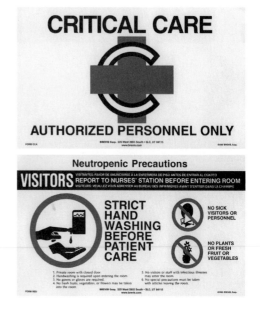

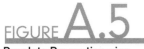

FIGURE A.5

Droplets Precaution sign

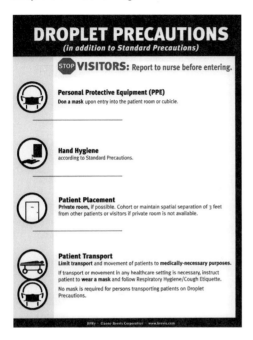

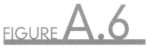

FIGURE A.6

Respiratory Hygiene sign

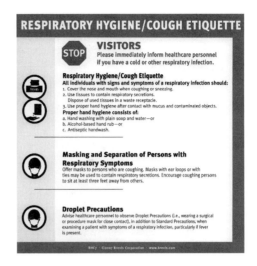

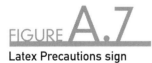

FIGURE A.7

Latex Precautions sign

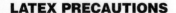
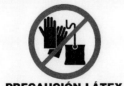

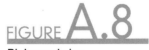

FIGURE A.8

Biohazard sign

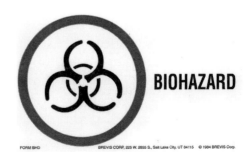

Additional Resources

1. Recommended Adult Immunization Schedule http://www.cdc.gov/mmwr/PDF/wk/mm5901-Immunization.pdf (pages 2–4 only)
2. Recommended Immunization Schedule for Persons Aged 0 Through 6 years http://www.cdc.gov/mmwr/PDF/wk/mm5851-Immunization.pdf (page 2 only)
3. Recommended Immunization Schedule for persons aged 7 through 18 years http://www.cdc.gov/mmwr/PDF/wk/mm5851-Immunization.pdf (page 3 only)
4. Catch-Up Immunization Schedule for persons aged 4 months through 18 years who start late or who are more than 1 month behind http://www.cdc.gov/mmwr/PDF/wk/mm5851-Immunization.pdf (page 4 only)
5. Guide to Contraindications and Precautions to Commonly Used Vaccines http://www.immunize.org/catg.d/p3072a.pdf
6. Hepatitis B Vaccine Information Statement http://www.immunize.org/vis/hepb01.pdf
7. H1N1 Vaccine Information Sheet http://www.immunize.org/vis/h1n1_inactiveflu.pdf
8. CDC Take 3 Actions to Fight the Flu http://www.cdc.gov/flu/freeresources/2009–10/pdf/take3_poster.pdf
9. Seasonal Influenza Vaccine Dosage Chart http://www.cdc.gov/flu/freeresources/2009–10/pdf/dosagechart.pdf
10. Disposing of Medical Sharps http://www.safeneedledisposal.org/assets/pdf/nursebroch.pdf
11. Traveling with Needles http://www.epa.gov/osw/nonhaz/industrial/medical/med-home.pdf
12. OSHA Log 300 http://www.osha.gov/recordkeeping/new-osha300form1-1-04.pdf page 7 of 12 only
13. If You Hear These Hoofbeats poster http://www.health.state.mn.us/bioterrorism/hcp/zebraanimal.pdf

Glossary

Acetaminophen

Medicine used to treat pain or fever. Sometimes called APAP.

Acquired immune deficiency syndrome (AIDS)

A disease of the human immune system caused by the human immunodeficiency virus.

Acquired in utero

Obtained while in mother's womb.

Active tuberculosis (TB) disease

A condition where tuberculosis bacteria (Mycobacterium tuberculosis) are multiplying and attacking a part of the body, usually the lungs. The most common symptoms of active TB disease include weakness, weight loss, fever, no appetite, chills, and sweating at night. A person with active TB disease may be infectious and spread TB bacteria to others.

Acute care hospital

A facility that is meant to treat patients with brief-but-severe episodes of illness, such as care given in an emergency room.

Acute HIV infection

Also known as primary HIV infection or acute retroviral syndrome (ARS). The period of rapid HIV replication that occurs 2 to 4 weeks after infection by HIV. Acute HIV infection is characterized by a drop in CD4 cell counts and an increase in HIV levels in the blood.

Advisory Committee on Immunization Practices (ACIP)

The ACIP consists of 15 experts in fields associated with immunization who have been selected by the Secretary of the U. S. Department of Health and Human Services to provide advice and guidance to the Secretary, the Assistant Secretary for Health, and the Centers for Disease Control and Prevention (CDC) on the control of vaccine-preventable diseases.

Airborne precautions

Procedures designed to reduce the risk of airborne transmission of infectious agents. Airborne transmission occurs by dissemination of airborne droplet nuclei or evaporated droplets that may remain suspended in the air for long periods of time, or dust particles containing the infectious agent. Microorganisms carried in this manner can be dispersed widely by air currents and may become inhaled by or deposited on a susceptible host within the same room or over a longer distance from the source patient, depending on environmental factors; therefore, special air handling and ventilation are required to prevent airborne transmission.

Airborne transmission	The transmission of microorganisms through the air, usually by a cough or sneeze.
Alcohol-based hand rub	An alcohol-containing preparation designed for application to the hands for reducing the number of viable microorganisms on the hands. In the United states, such preparations usually contain 60% to 95% ethanol or isopropanol.
American Academy of Family Physicians (AAFP)	A large national medical organization representing family physicians, family medicine residents, and medical students nationwide.
American Academy of Pediatrics (AAP)	A large national medical association of pediatricians committed to the attainment of optimal physical, mental, and social health and well-being for all infants, children, adolescents, and young adults.
Anorexia	Lack of desire to eat.
Antibiotic resistance	When an antibiotic drug has no effect on a microorganism.
Antibodies	Also known as immunoglobulins. Antibodies are produced in the body and are found in blood and body fluids. Antibodies are produced to neutralize and remove bacteria.
Antifungal	Opposes or interferes with replication of a fungus.
Antigen	A molecule that binds with an individual antibody.
Antimicrobial	Opposes or interferes with replication of a microbe.
Antipyretic	Medication that reduces body temperature during a fever.
Antisepsis	The destruction of microorganisms on living tissue.
Antiseptic	A chemical agent used in antisepsis.
Antitoxin	An antibody preparation that can neutralize a specific toxin.
Antivirals	Opposes or interferes with replication of a virus.
Arthralgia	Severe pain in a joint.
Ascites	Fluid build up in the abdomen, which can be caused by liver damage, heart failure, malnutrition, or infection.
Aseptic	Preventing infection.
Asymptomatic	When a patient carries a disease or infection but experiences no symptoms.

Atelectasis A lung condition in which the alveoli are deflated, causing a lack of gas exchange.

Bacillus Calmette-Guérin (BCG) A live vaccine against the tuberculosis bacteria. BCG is rarely used in the United States, but it is often given to infants and small children in other countries where tuberculosis is common.

Bacteremia Bacterial infection in the bloodstream.

Bacteria A living microorganism that can produce disease in a host.

Benchmarks A standard by which something can be measured or judged.

Biofilm A group of microorganisms that has become stuck together and/or to a surface.

Biohazard container A puncture-resistant box used for the disposal of contaminated needles, sharps, and other infectious materials.

Bioterrorism A form of terrorism that involves the intentional release of potentially harmful biological agents, such as bacteria, viruses, and toxins.

Bloodborne precautions Procedures designed to minimize the transmission of disease through blood or other body fluids. Pathogenic microorganisms that may be present in human blood or other potentially infected materials can infect and cause disease in persons who are exposed to blood containing the pathogen. These pathogens include, but are not limited to, hepatitis B virus (HBV), hepatitis C virus (HCV), and human immunodeficiency virus (HIV). Bloodborne pathogens are spread through percutaneous or mucocutaneous exposure with contaminated blood and bodily fluids.

Bloodborne transmission Transmission of a disease agent by blood contaminated with the agent.

Botulism Severe paralysis of the muscles caused by the botulinum toxin of the bacterium *Clostridium botulinum*.

Broad-spectrum antibiotics An antibiotic with activity against a wide range of disease-causing bacteria. It commonly refers to antibiotics that act against both Gram-positive and Gram-negative bacteria.

Bubonic/buboes Buboes are enlarged lymph nodes, or swollen glands. The bubonic plague refers to the swollen glands in the groin.

Burn unit A hospital area that is used specifically to care for patients who have sustained burns.

Carbapenemase An enzyme that can inactivate the effects of an antimicrobial agent.

Carcinogen	Any cancer-causing substance or agent.
Catarrhal	Relating to the inflammation of a mucous membrane, typically of the sinus and throat.
Centers for Disease Control and Prevention (CDC)	A government agency dedicated to protecting health and promoting quality of life through the prevention and control of disease, injury, and disability.
Centers for Medicare and Medicaid Services (CMS)	A division of the U.S. Department of Health and Human Services that ensures effective, up-to-date health care coverage and promotes quality care for beneficiaries.
Chest x-ray	A picture of the heart, lungs, airways, blood vessels, and the bones of the spine. A chest x-ray is made by exposing a film to x-rays that pass through the chest.
Circulating nurse	A nurse who monitors a surgical procedure, ensuring that operating room conditions remain sterile and safe for the patient. Presurgical setup and surgery-related paperwork are also often duties of the circulating nurse.
Cirrhosis	A type of chronic liver disease.
Cleaning	The removal of visible soil.
Clean-up operation	A procedure where-by hazardous substances are removed, contained, incinerated, neutralized, stabilized, cleared-up, or in any other manner processed or handled with the ultimate goal of making the site safer for people or the environment.
Closed gloving	A technique that requires the surgical staff to insert arms into, but not through, the sleeves of the gown, and to wait for an assistant to pull the gown over the shoulders. The surgical staff must then use their hands within the cuffs to put gloves on without touching the gloves with bare hands.
Colonization	The presence and multiplication of microorganisms without actual tissue invasion, damage, or infection.
Communicable disease	An infection that is capable of being easily communicated or transmitted from one person to another person.
Communicable period	The time after an infection when the infectious agent may be transmitted to another host.
Complement System	A component of the immune system that helps eliminate pathogens from the body.
Conjunctivitis	Inflammation of the conjunctiva of the eye, sometimes called "pink-eye."
Contact precautions	Procedures designed to reduce the risk of transmission of epidemiologically important microorganisms by direct

or indirect contact. Direct-contact transmission involves skin-to-skin contact and physical transfer of microorganisms to a susceptible host from an infected or colonized person, such as occurs when personnel turn patients, bathe patients, or perform other patient-care activities that require physical contact. Direct-contact transmission also can occur between two patients, with one serving as the source of infectious microorganisms and the other as a susceptible host. Indirect-contact transmission involves contact of a susceptible host with a contaminated intermediate object, usually inanimate, in the patient's environment. Contact precautions apply to specified patients known or suspected to be infected or colonized with epidemiologically important microorganisms that can be transmitted by direct or indirect contact.

Contact transmission	Transmission of a disease agent by direct physical contact with the agent.
Contagion	The direct cause of a communicable disease.
Coronary care unit (CCU)	A specialized area of a hospital that cares for patients with cardiac conditions.
Critical items	Any item that enters sterile tissue or the vascular system. These items are at high risk of transmitting infection if contaminated, and must be sterile.
Cyanosis	Bluing of the skin, lips, gums, and nailbeds, caused by lack of oxygen.
Decontamination	The removal of hazardous substances from employees and their equipment to the extent necessary to preclude the occurrence of foreseeable adverse health affects.
Decubitis ulcer	A chronic wound or ulcer on the skin and subcutaneous tissues, acquired from prolonged pressure on one part of the body for an extended period of time; also known as a bedsore.
Denominator	The number written below the line in a common fraction that indicates the number of parts into which one whole is.
Dependent variable	Factor that is being measured in an experiment and what is affected during the experiment.
Dialysis catheter	Tubing used for exchanging blood to and from the hemodialysis machine from the patient.
Diaphragm	A muscle that allows the chest to move air in and out of the lungs.

Direct transmission	Transmission of a disease from one person to another through direct contact with infected blood, body fluids, or other infectious material.
Directly observed therapy (DOT)	A method used to ensure adherence with medications. The patient meets with a health care worker every day or several times a week and takes the medicine while the health care worker watches.
Disinfection	The elimination of many or all pathogenic microorganisms except bacterial spores.
Droplet precautions	Procedures designed to reduce the risk of droplet transmission of infectious agents. Droplet transmission involves contact of the conjunctivae or the mucous membranes of the nose or mouth of a susceptible person with large-particle droplets (larger than 5 um in size) containing microorganisms generated from a person who has a clinical disease or who is a carrier of the microorganism. Droplets are generated from the source person primarily during coughing, sneezing, or talking and during the performance of certain procedures such as suctioning and bronchoscopy. Transmission via large-particle droplets requires close contact between source and recipient persons.
Dyspnea	Difficulty breathing.
Emergency response	An effort by employees from outside the immediate release area or by other designated responders to an occurrence that results, or is likely to result, in an uncontrolled release of a hazardous substance.
Encephalitis	Neurological disorder characterized by inflammation of the brain. Common symptoms include headaches, fevers, drowsiness, hyperactivity, and/or general weakness.
Encephalopathy	Any diffuse disease of the brain that alters brain function or structure. Can be caused by bacteria or virus metabolic or mitochondrial dysfunction, brain tumor or increased pressure in the skull, prolonged exposure to a toxin, chronic progressive trauma, poor nutrition, or lack of oxygen or blood flow to the brain. The hallmark of encephalopathy is an altered mental state.
Endogenous	Microorganisms from patient's normal flora.
Endometritis	Inflammation of the endometrium or the inner lining of the uterus.
Endotracheal intubation	Insertion of a tube into the trachea for purposes of anesthesia, airway maintenance, aspiration of secretions, lung ventilation, or prevention of entrance of foreign material into the airway.

Environmental hygiene Sanitation of public areas.

Epidemiology The branch of medicine that deals with the study of the causes, distribution, and control of disease in populations.

Epiglottitis Severe swelling of the throat structures that make it difficult to swallow and breathe.

Eschar A dry scabbed area of skin that forms after cauterization or burning.

Ethambutol An antibiotic used in the treatment of tuberculosis.

Exogenous From the environment or from outside the organism or system.

Exposure Contact with blood, body fluids, or potentially infectious material.

Extensively drug-resistant TB A rare type of tuberculosis disease that is caused by a strain of *Mycobacterium tuberculosis* that is resistant to nearly all medicines commonly used to treat tuberculosis.

Extrapulmonary TB Active tuberculosis disease in any part of the body other than the lung, such as the kidney, spine, brain, or lymph nodes.

False negative A test result of negative, but in actuality the variable being measured is there, and the test should have been positive.

False positive A test result of positive, but in actuality the variable being measured is not there, and the test should have been negative.

Fasciitis A rapidly progressive inflammatory disease that destroys muscles, fat, and skin tissue.

Fatigue A tired state.

Fecal–oral route The spread of infection from stool to mouth.

Fish bone analysis A method of systematically looking at effects and the causes that create or contribute to those effects. Because of the function of the fish bone analysis, it may be referred to as a cause-and-effect analysis. The design of the diagram used in the analysis looks much like the skeleton of a fish, and therefore, it is often referred to as the fish bone diagram.

Fit test A procedure that is performed to determine the correct size of a particulate respirator, for example, an N95 mask, for a particular person.

Flaccid paralysis An effect of muscular nerve damage in which muscle tone is weakened or lost.

Fomites An inanimate object (as a dish, toy, book, doorknob, or clothing) that may become contaminated with infectious organisms and serve in their transmission.

Germicidal	Any germ-killing agent or disinfectant.
Granulomata	Tumors that result when the skin that forms over a wound becomes inflamed or infected. The plural of granuloma.
Growth Factor	Chemical that stimulates cell growth.
Guillain-Barré Syndrome (GBS)	A disease of the nervous system that causes muscle weakness, loss of reflexes, and numbness or tingling in the arms, legs, face, and other parts of the body.
Hand hygiene and washing	The practice of cleansing the hands of pathogens and chemicals that can cause harm to patients. Hands must be washed with antimicrobial soap and water for 15 to 20 seconds. Use of an alcohol rub is also an acceptable hand hygiene practice in selected clinical situations.
Hazardous materials response (HAZMAT) team	An organized group of employees, typically designated by the employer, who are expected to perform work to handle and control actual or potential leaks or spills of hazardous substances requiring possible close approach to the substance. The team members perform responses to releases or potential releases of hazardous substances for the purpose of control or stabilization of the incident. A HAZMAT team is not a fire brigade, nor is a typical fire brigade a HAZMAT team. A HAZMAT team, however, may be a separate component of a fire brigade or fire department.
Hazardous waste	Any substance, biological agent, or disease causing agent that when released into the environment and upon exposure, ingestion, inhalation, or assimilation into any person may result in adverse effects on the health or safety of individuals either directly from the environment or indirectly by ingestion through food chains. Hazardous waste will or may reasonably be anticipated to cause death, disease, behavioral abnormalities, cancer, genetic mutation, physiological malfunctions, or physical deformations in exposed persons or their offspring.
Health care–associated infection	Infection acquired in a health care facility; also known as nosocomial infection.
Health hazard	A chemical, mixture of chemicals, or a pathogen that may cause acute or chronic health effects to occur in exposed employees. The term *health hazard* includes chemicals that are carcinogens, toxic or highly toxic agents, reproductive toxins, irritants, corrosives, sensitizers, hepatotoxins, nephrotoxins, neurotoxins, agents that act on the hematopoietic system, and agents that damage the lungs, skin, eyes, or mucous membranes. It also includes stress due to temperature extremes.

Hematoma	Leakage of blood from a vessel into surrounding tissues that forms a hard, painful, black and blue collection of blood under the skin.
Hematopoietic	Pertaining to the formation of blood or blood cells.
Hematuria	The presence of blood in the urine, indicative of kidney disease or urinary tract infection.
Hemorrhage	Loss of blood.
Hepatitis A virus	Hepatitis A virus typically causes an infection in the liver. Hepatitis A virus infection produces a self-limited disease that does not result in chronic infection or chronic liver disease. Hepatitis A virus infection is primarily transmitted by the fecal–oral route, by either person-to-person contact or through consumption of contaminated food or water.
Hepatitis B virus	Hepatitis B virus typically causes an infection in the liver. It can range in severity from a mild illness lasting a few weeks to a serious, lifelong illness. Hepatitis B is usually spread when blood, semen, or another body fluid from a person infected with the Hepatitis B virus enters the body of someone who is not infected. This can happen through sexual contact with an infected person or sharing needles, syringes, or other drug-injection equipment. Hepatitis B can also be passed from an infected mother to her baby at birth.
Hepatitis C virus	Hepatitis C virus typically causes an infection in the liver. This infection is the most common chronic bloodborne infection in the United States. Although HCV is not efficiently transmitted sexually, persons at risk for infection through injection drug use might seek care in STD treatment facilities, HIV counseling and testing facilities, correctional facilities, drug treatment facilities, and other public health settings where STD and HIV prevention and control services are available.
Herd immunity	Type of immunity that occurs when the vaccination of a portion of the population (or herd) provides protection to unprotected individuals.
High-efficiency particulate air (HEPA)	A filter designed to remove 99.97% of airborne particles measuring 0.3 micrometers or greater in diameter.
High touch area	A surface that is more likely to harbor microscopic germs due to frequent contact with human skin. Doorknobs, drinking fountains, and computer keyboards are examples of high touch areas.

Histogram	A display of statistical information that uses rectangles to graphically show the frequency of data items.
Home care	The delivery of health care in the home setting.
Human immunodefi-ciency virus (HIV)	The virus that causes AIDS.
Hyperbaric	High pressure, usually used in reference to oxygen.
Immediately Dangerous to Life or Health (IDLH)	An atmospheric concentration of any toxic, corrosive, or as-phyxiant substance that poses an immediate threat to life, or would cause irreversible or delayed adverse health effects, or would interfere with an individual's ability to escape from a dangerous atmosphere.
Immunity	The resistance of a host to an infectious agent.
Immunization	Administering a vaccine to prevent disease.
Immunosuppressed	Suppression of the immune response, as by drugs or radiation, in order to prevent the rejection of grafts or transplants or to control autoimmune diseases.
Independent variable	A factor that can be varied or manipulated in an experiment (e.g., time, temperature, concentration, etc.).
Indirect transmission	Transmission of a disease from one person to another without direct contact.
Induration	Size and mobility of a palpable mass; a palpable, raised, hardened area.
Influenza	A highly contagious viral infection of the nose, throat, and lungs. It is one of the most severe illnesses of the winter season and spreads easily when an infected person coughs or sneezes. Influenza may lead to hospitalization or even death. Typical symptoms include a sudden high fever, chills, a dry cough, headache, runny nose, sore throat, and muscle and joint pain.
Inherited immunity	To receive from one's parents by genetic transmission resistance to infection by a specific pathogen.
Intensivist	An intensive care specialist.
Intradermal	Administration of medication or immunization between the layers of the skin.
Intubation	Placement of a tube into an external or internal orifice of the body. Most commonly refers to endotracheal intubation or placement of a flexible plastic tube into the trachea to protect the patient's airway and provide a means of mechanical ventilation.
Intussusception	The enfolding of a part of the intestine within another part of the intestine.
Isolation room	A room for patients with highly communicable diseases.

Jaundice	A yellow color to skin.
Laceration	A roughly torn area of tissue, distinct from a cut or incision.
Laryngospasm	The sudden inability of the vocal cord muscles to move properly.
Latent tuberculosis (TB) disease	A condition in which Mycobacterium tuberculosis bacteria are alive but inactive in the body. In patients with latent tuberculosis infection, there are no symptoms and they cannot spread the infection, but they usually have a positive skin test reaction. These patients may develop active tuberculosis disease at a later time if treatment for latent tuberculosis infection is not initiated.
Live, attenuated influenza vaccine	Vaccines prepared from attenuated strains that are almost or completely devoid of pathogenicity but are capable of inducing a protective immune response.
Lockjaw	Spasm of the jaw muscles resulting in unrestrained muscle fire and sustained muscular contraction; also known as tetanus.
Long-term care facilities	A nursing home for patients that provides 24 hour, 7 days a week chronic or long-term nursing care and medical treatment. Typically used for more stable patients.
Malaise	A generalized feeling of bodily discomfort and fatigue.
Mantoux test	A diagnostic tool for tuberculosis; the intradermal injection of tuberculin bacteria to determine prescence of infection.
Mastitis	Infection of the breast.
Mean	The mathematical average of all the terms. To calculate it, the values of all the terms are added and then divided by the number of terms.
Mechanical Ventilation	A form of respiratory support that delivers oxygen by a machine that moves air in and out of the lungs.
Median	The value of a group of numbers such that the number of terms having values greater than or equal to it is the same as the number of terms having values less than or equal to it. If the number of terms is odd, then the median is the value of the term in the middle. If the number of terms is even, then the median is the average of the two terms in the middle, such that the number of terms having values greater than or equal to it is the same as the number of terms having values less than or equal to it.
Medicaid	The U.S. government's health insurance program for low-income individuals and families who fit into an eligibility group. Medicaid is a state-administered program, and each state sets its own guidelines regarding eligibility and services.

Medical waste	All waste materials generated at health care facilities, such as hospitals, clinics, physician's offices, dental practices, blood banks, and veterinary hospitals/clinics, as well as medical research facilities and laboratories. This includes any waste that is generated in the diagnosis, treatment, or immunization of human beings or animals, in research pertaining thereto, or in the production or testing of biologicals.
Medicare	The U.S. government's health insurance program for elderly and disabled Americans.
Meningitis	Disease caused by the inflammation of the protective membranes covering the brain and spinal cord known as the meninges. The inflammation is usually caused by an infection, either bacterial, viral, or fungal, of the fluid surrounding the brain and spinal cord.
Miliary tuberculosis (TB)	A disease caused by the bacteria *Mycobacterium tuberculosis,* where the bacteria is disseminated and affects many organs.
Mode	The most frequently occurring value in a frequency distribution.
Mode of transmission	The method by which a disease or infection is transferred.
Morbidity	The relative incidence of a particular disease in a specific population.
Mortality	The relative frequency of deaths in a specific population; death rate.
Multidrug-resistant tuberculosis (MDR TB)	Active TB disease caused by bacteria resistant to two or more of the most important medicines such as isoniazid and rifampin.
Myalgia	Muscle aches.
N95 respirator	The most common type of particulate filtering facepiece respirators. Filters at least 95% of airborne particles but is not resistant to oil.
Necrotic	Tissue that has died due to disease or injury.
Needleless intravenous (IV) tubing systems	Intravenous tubing that does not require a needle to administer medications. Designed to reduce the incidence of needlestick injuries.
Negative	Usually refers to a test result. For example, a negative tuberculosis test means that the patient does not have tuberculosis.
Neutropenia	An abnormal decrease in the number of neutrophils in the blood.

Neutropenic precautions	A procedure whereby the health care personnel utilize strict isolation procedures and techniques in order to prevent infection in a patient with a low neutrophil count.
Noncritical items	Any item that may come into contact with intact skin, but not mucous membranes. Sterility of these items is considered noncritical.
Nonproductive cough	To expel air from the lungs suddenly with a harsh noise, often involuntarily without expelling secretions.
Normal distribution	A pattern for the distribution of a set of data that follows a bell-shaped curve. The bell shape is concentrated in the center and decreases on either side. This means that the data has less of a tendency to produce unusually extreme values compared to some other distributions. The bell-shaped curve is symmetric. This means the probability of deviations from the mean are comparable in either direction. Also called the Gaussian distribution.
Nosocomial	Infection originating in a hospital.
Numerator	The expression written above the line in a common fraction to indicate the number of parts of the whole.
Occupational exposure	When an employee has come in contact with a potential communicable disease while performing a task in the workplace.
Occupational Safety and Health Administration (OSHA)	A division of the U. S. Department of Labor that ensures safe and healthful working conditions for working individuals.
Oliguria	Diminished production and excretion of urine.
Omphalitis	An inflammation of the umbilical area.
Open gloving	The technique of putting gloves on with clean, bare hands.
Opportunistic pathogen	Any pathogen that is generally harmless when it exists in the human body unless the host's immune system becomes impaired.
Opthalmia neonatorum	A form of conjunctivitis that occurs within the first 10 days of life, typically as a result of contact with infected vaginal discharge from the birth canal.
Orchitis	Inflammation of the testis.
Otitis media	Infection of the middle ear or tympanic membrane.
Papular	An area of tissue that has developed papules, or small raised areas.
Parotitis	Swelling of the parotid or salivary glands, commonly seen in mumps infection.
Paroxysmal	Related to a sudden outburst or intensification of symptoms such as cough.

Pathogen	A microorganism capable of producing disease.
Pediatric intensive care unit (PICU)	A specialized hospital unit in which the patients, age birth to 17 years, require specialized care, and the nurse–patient ratio is low.
Percutaneous	Through the skin or using a very small incision.
Pericardium	Thin sac that surrounds the heart and the roots of the great blood vessels.
Permissible exposure limit (PEL)	The exposure, inhalation, or dermal permissible exposure limit specified in 29 CFR part 1910, subparts G and Z. Published exposure level means the exposure limits published in *NIOSH Recommendations for Occupational Health Standards,* dated 1986, which is incorporated by reference as specified in § 1910.6 or if none is specified, the exposure limits published in the standards specified by the American Conference of Governmental Industrial Hygienists in their publication *Threshold Limit Values and Biological Exposure Indices for 1987–88,* dated 1987, which is incorporated by reference as specified in § 1910.6.
Personal protective equipment (PPE)	Type of dress designed to protect employees from serious workplace injuries or illnesses resulting from contact with chemical, radiological, physical, electrical, mechanical, or other workplace hazards. Besides face shields, safety glasses, hard hats, and safety shoes, PPE can include a variety of devices and garments, such as goggles, coveralls, gloves, vests, earplugs, and respirators.
Pharyngitis	Inflammation of the throat. Also known as sore throat.
Plague	A disease that is transferred to humans through the bites of infected rodent fleas.
Plasmid	A gene carrier molecule, most commonly found in bacteria, that is separate from the chromosomal DNA.
Pleurisy	Inflammation of the pleura, or the moist, double-layered membrane that surrounds the lungs and lines the rib cage. Also called pleuritis.
Pneumonia	An infection of the lungs that can be caused by nearly any known class of infection-causing organisms.
Pneumonic	Pertaining to the lungs, or pertaining to pneumonia.
Polysaccharide	A sugar coating that is usually found as part of cells and their components.
Positive	Usually refers to a medical test result. For example, if you have a positive tuberculosis skin test reaction, you likely are infected with the tuberculosis bacteria.

Post emergency response	That portion of an emergency response performed after the immediate threat of a release has been stabilized or eliminated and clean up of the site has begun.
Postherpetic neuralgia (PHN)	Persistent burning and hypersensitivity of a cutaneous nerve in an area following an attack of herpes zoster.
Precautions	The constellation of activities intended to minimize exposure to an infectious agent; precautions imply the isolation of an infected patient.
Prospective	Relating to the future.
Prophylaxis	Any measure taken to prevent a disease or condition.
Prospective payment system (PPS)	Method of reimbursement in which Medicare payment is made based on a predetermined, fixed amount. The payment amount for a particular service is derived based on the classification system of that service (for example, diagnosis-related groups for inpatient hospital services).
Proteinaceous material	A thick, slimy, gel-like material that contains protein.
Proton pump inhibitor (PPI)	A group of medicine that blocks the acid-producing enzyme in the wall of the stomach.
Pseudomembranous colitis	Severe inflammation of the inner lining of the colon.
Pulmonary	Relating to the lungs.
Pulmonary TB	The most active tuberculosis disease that occurs in the lungs.
Purified protein derivative (PPD)	Diagnostic aid used to detect mycobacterium tuberculosis. Injected intradermally.
Pyelonephritis	A kidney infection that is usually caused by bacteria that ascends from the bladder, through the ureters, up to the kidneys.
Pyrazinamide	Medication used in treatment of tuberculosis.
Qualified person	A person with specific training, knowledge, and experience in the area for which the person has the responsibility and the authority to control. For example, site safety and health supervisor (or official) means the individual located on a hazardous waste site who is responsible to the employer and has the authority and knowledge necessary to implement the site safety and health plan and verify compliance with applicable safety and health requirements.

QuantiFERON-TB Gold or QFT test	QuantiFERON®-TB Gold is an *in vitro* laboratory diagnostic test using a whole blood specimen. It is an indirect test for *M. tuberculosis* complex (i.e., *M. tuberculosis, M. bovis, M. africanum, M. microti, M. canetti*) infection, whether active tuberculosis disease or latent tuberculosis infection.
Rank order	An arrangement according to rank.
Resistant bacteria	Bacteria that can no longer be killed by certain antibiotics.
Retrospective	Relating to the past.
Rhinitis	Irritation and inflammation of internal areas of the nose. The primary symptom of rhinitis is nasal dripping. It is caused by chronic or acute inflammation of the mucous membrane of the nose due to viruses, bacteria, or irritants.
Rhinorrhea	A runny nose.
Ribosome	The essential protein producer of a cell, located in the cytoplasm.
Rigors	Shaking chills.
Root cause analysis	Procedure for analyzing the causes of operations problems in an effort to determine what can be done to solve or prevent them.
Secondary bacterial infection	A bacterial infection that develops after an initial inflammatory event, usually a viral infection.
Semicritical items	Any item that comes into contact with a mucous membrane or nonintact skin. These items must be disinfected with high-level chemical disinfectants.
Septicemia	A life-threatening blood infection that occurs when bacteria enter the bloodstream.
Seroconversion	A change in the blood test levels from a negative to a positive result.
Sharps	Any device with corners, edges, or projections capable of cutting or piercing the skin.
Sharps container	A puncture-resistant, leak-proof biohazard container that is used for the safe disposal of needles, syringes, and scalpels. The container can be stationary or transportable.
Shingles	A skin rash caused by the Varicella zoster virus. It occurs among people who have previously contracted the virus, such as people who have had the chickenpox, and the reactivation of the virus can be due to stress or immune system deficiency.
Single-lumen power implanted subcutaneous power port	A type of intravenous catheter used for administration of medications, blood or blood products, or intravenous infusions.

Single-lumen subcutaneously implanted port	A type of intravenous catheter with one opening that is used for administration of medications, blood or blood products, or intravenous infusions.
Small quantity generator	A generator of hazardous wastes that in any calendar month generates no more than 1,000 kilograms (2,205 pounds) of hazardous waste in that month.
Smear	A test to see whether there are tuberculosis bacteria in sputum.
Sodium hypochlorite	A chemical compound (sodium, oxygen, chlorine) that is used in bleach and disinfectant.
Souring	The addition of acid to correct the pH of a solution. Used in the laundering process to eliminate alkalinity and preserve fabric integrity.
Sphygmomanometer	Instrumentation used to measure blood pressure that consists of an air pump and a gauge attached to a rubber cuff that wraps around the upper arm.
Spill	An inadvertent release of a liquid usually regarded as hazardous to human health.
Spores	A walled, single- to many-celled, reproductive body of an organism, capable of giving rise to a new individual either directly or indirectly; a germ, germ cell, or seed. Spores are not inactivated when using alcohol-based hand rubs. Hand washing with an antimicrobial soap and water is required.
Sputum	Phlegm coughed up from deep inside the lungs. Sputum is examined for TB bacteria using a smear; part of the sputum can also be used to do a culture.
Standard Precautions	Procedures designed to reduce transmission of bloodborne pathogens. Standard precautions assume that all patients are infectious, and apply to blood, all body fluids, secretions, excretions (except sweat), nonintact skin, and mucous membranes whether or not blood is visible. The procedures call for: (1) handwashing between patient contact; (2) gloves when touching blood, body fluids, excretions, secretions, or contaminated items; (3) mask, eye protection, and gowns if the patient care activity may result in splashes or sprays of blood or secretions/excretions; (4) careful handling of patient equipment and linen to reduce transmission and environmental contamination; (5) avoiding exposure to needles and sharps; and (6) use of mouthpieces and resuscitation bags when necessary.
Sterilization	The elimination of all forms of microbial life.
Stridor	A harsh noise caused by inhaling through a constricted airway.

Subglottal	Relating to the lower part of the larynx that runs between the vocal cords and the trachea.
Surgical hand scrub	An antiseptic-containing preparation used by surgical personnel to eliminate transient and reduce resident hand flora.
Surgical intensive care unit (SICU)	A post-operative unit of a hospital whereby the patient requires specialized care and the nurse–patient ratio is low.
Susceptibility tests	Exam to determine the lack of ability to resist extraneous agents, such as a pathogen or drug.
Susceptible	When an individual is at risk for infection.
Tachycardia	Rapid heart rate.
Tachypnia	Rapid breathing.
Terminal disinfection	The disinfection of the area occupied by a patient once the patient is no longer a source of infection, or is deceased.
Thrombocytopenia	A platelet deficiency.
TORCH	Acronym for infections passed from a pregnant woman to her fetus: Toxoplasma, Other (hepatitis B, syphilis, Varicella-zoster virus, HIV, parvovirus B19), Rubella, Cytomegalovirus, Herpes simplex.
Toxic megacolon	A complication of inflammatory bowel disease in which the rapid dilation of the large intestine can cause the colon to tear; it is life threatening if left untreated.
Toxin	A poison produced by an organism, characterized by antigenicity in certain animals and high molecular weight, and including the bacterial toxins that are the causative agents of tetanus, diphtheria, etc., and such plant and animal toxins as ricin and snake venom.
Transmission	The spread of an infecting agent to another host.
Transmission-based precautions	Procedures designed for patients documented or suspected to be infected with highly transmissible or epidemiologically important pathogens for which additional precautions beyond standard precautions are needed to interrupt transmission in hospitals. There are three types of transmission-based precautions: airborne precautions, droplet precautions, and contact precautions. They may be combined for diseases that have multiple routes of transmission. When used either singularly or in combination, they are to be used in addition to standard precautions.
Triple-lumen power PICC	A type of intravenous catheter with three ports that is used for administration of medications, blood or blood products, or intravenous infusions.

Triple-lumen short-term central venous catheter (CVC)	A type of intravenous catheter with three openings that is used for administration of medications, blood or blood products, or intravenous infusions.
Tuberculin or PPD	A liquid that is injected under the skin on the lower part of the arm during a tuberculosis skin test.
Tuberculin blood test	A new test that uses a blood sample to find out if you are infected with tuberculosis bacteria. The test measures the response to TB proteins when they are mixed with a small amount of blood. Examples of these special TB blood tests include QuantiFERON®-TB Gold (QFT-G) and T-Spot®.*TB* test.
Tuberculin skin test (TST)	A test that is often used to find out if infection with the tuberculosis bacteria is present. A liquid called tuberculin is injected under the skin on the lower part of the arm.
Uncontrolled hazardous waste site	An area identified as an uncontrolled hazardous waste site by a governmental body, whether federal, state, local, or other, where an accumulation of hazardous substances creates a threat to the health and safety of individuals, the environment, or both. Some sites are found on public lands such as those created by former municipal, county, or state landfills where illegal or poorly managed waste disposal has taken place. Other sites are found on private property, often belonging to generators or former generators of hazardous substance wastes. Examples of such sites include, but are not limited to, surface impoundments, landfills, dumps, and tank or drum farms.
Urosepsis	A urinary tract infection invading the bloodstream and causing sepsis.
Vaccine	A biological preparation that provokes or improves immunity to a specific disease.
Vaccine information statement (VIS)	Information sheets produced by the Centers for Disease Control and Prevention (CDC). VISs explain both the benefits and risks of a vaccine to adult vaccine recipients and the parents or legal representatives of vaccines who are children and adolescents. Federal law requires that VISs be handed out whenever certain vaccinations are given (before each dose).
Vascular access	A means of gaining entry to a patient's bloodstream. There are three types of vascular access: a fistula connects a patient's artery with a vein (surgically); a graft connects a patient's artery and vein with a piece of artificial vein; and a catheter is a plastic tube inserted into a central vein.
Vegetative pathogen	Bacteria that does not form spores; vegetative bacteria is less resistant to heating processes than spore-forming bacteria.

Ventilator	A machine that assists patients with respiratory gas exchange, also known as an artificial respirator.
Ventilator acquired pneumonia (VAP)	A type of bacteria in the lungs that a patient develops while on a breathing machine.
Vesicle	Any small anatomical pouch, or a small blister on skin or on a mucous membrane.
Visibly soiled hands	Hands showing visible dirt or that are visibly contaminated with proteinaceous material, blood, or other body fluids.
Waterless antiseptic agent	An antiseptic agent that does not require the use of exogenous water. After applying such an agent, the hands are rubbed together until the agent has dried.
Wheal	Small raised area on the skin.

Index